T0259123

Cardiac Implantable Electronic Devices and Congenital Heart Disease

Editors

CHEYENNE M. BEACH
MAULLY J. SHAH

CARDIAC ELECTROPHYSIOLOGY CLINICS

www.cardiacEP.theclinics.com

Consulting Editors
EMILY P. ZEITLER
LUIGI DI BIASE

December 2023 • Volume 15 • Number 4

ELSEVIER

1600 John F. Kennedy Boulevard • Suite 1800 • Philadelphia, Pennsylvania, 19103-2899

http://www.theclinics.com

CARDIAC ELECTROPHYSIOLOGY CLINICS Volume 15, Number 4
December 2023 ISSN 1877-9182, ISBN-13: 978-0-443-18415-4

Editor: Joanna Gascoine
Developmental Editor: Shivank Joshi

Cardiac Electrophysiology Clinics (ISSN 1877-9182) is published quarterly by Elsevier Inc., 360 Park Avenue South, New York, NY 10010-1710. Months of issue are March, June, September, and December. Subscription prices are $259.00 per year for US individuals, $464.00 per year for US institutions, $272.00 per year for Canadian individuals, $524.00 per year for Canadian institutions, $331.00 per year for international individuals, $562.00 per year for international institutions and $100.00 per year for US, Canadian and international students/residents. To receive student/resident rate, orders must be accompanied by name of affiliated institution, date of term, and the signature of program/residency coordinator on institution letterhead. Orders will be billed at individual rate until proof of status is received. Foreign air speed delivery is included in all Clinics subscription prices. All prices are subject to change without notice. **POSTMASTER:** Send address changes to Cardiac Electrophysiology Clinics, Elsevier Health Sciences Division, Subscription Customer Service, 3251 Riverport Lane, Maryland Heights, MO 63043. **Customer Service: 1-800-654-2452 (US and Canada). From outside of the US and Canada, call 314-477-8871. Fax: 314-447-8029. E-mail: JournalsCustomerService-usa@elsevier.com (for print support); JournalsOnlineSupport-usa@elsevier.com (for online support).**

Reprints. For copies of 100 or more of articles in this publication, please contact the Commercial Reprints Department, Elsevier Inc., 360 Park Avenue South, New York, NY 10010-1710. Tel.: 212-633-3874; Fax: 212-633-3820; E-mail: reprints@elsevier.com.

Cardiac Electrophysiology Clinics is covered in MEDLINE/PubMed (Index Medicus).

Contributors

CONSULTING EDITORS

EMILY P. ZEITLER, MD, MHS, FHRS
Cardiac Electrophysiology Assistant Prof of Medicine, Geisel School of Medicine, Hanover, New Hampshire, USA; Assistant Prof of Health Care Policy, The Dartmouth Institute Dartmouth-Hitchcock Medical Center, Lebanon, New Hampshire, USA

LUIGI DI BIASE, MD, MHS, FHRS
Section Head of Electrophysiology Director of Arrhythmia Services Professor of Medicine (Cardiology) Montefiore-Einstein Center for Heart and Vascular Care, Montefiore Medical Center, Albert Einstein College of Medicine, Bronx, New York, USA

EDITORS

CHEYENNE M. BEACH, MD, CEPS-P
Associate Professor, Department of Pediatrics, Section of Pediatric Cardiology, Yale School of Medicine, New Haven, Connecticut, USA

MAULLY J. SHAH, MBBS, FACC, FHRS, CCDS, CEPS
Professor of Pediatrics, Director of Cardiac Electrophysiology, The Children's Hospital of Philadelphia, Perelman School of Medicine, University of Pennsylvania, Philadelphia, Pennsylvania, USA; Professor of Pediatrics, Division of Pediatric Cardiology, Children's National Hospital, Division of Cardiology Washington, Washington DC, USA

AUTHORS

CHEYENNE M. BEACH, MD, CEPS-P
Associate Professor, Department of Pediatrics, Section of Pediatric Cardiology, Yale School of Medicine, New Haven, Connecticut, USA

CHARLES I. BERUL, MD
Division of Pediatric Cardiology, Department of Pediatrics, Masonic Children's Hospital, University of Minnesota Medical School, Minneapolis, Minnesota, USA; Division of Cardiology, Department of Pediatrics, Children's National Hospital, George Washington University School of Medicine, Washington, DC, USA

ANICA BULIC, MD
Assistant Professor of Paediatrics, University of Toronto, The Hospital for Sick Children, Labatt Family Heart Centre, Toronto, Ontario, Canada

HENRY CHUBB, MA, MBBS, PhD, FHRS
Clinical Assistant Professor, Stanford University School of Medicine, Stanford Medicine Children's Health, Pediatric Heart Center, Palo Alto, California, USA

BRADLEY C. CLARK, MD
Division of Pediatric Cardiology, Department of Pediatrics, Masonic Children's Hospital, University of Minnesota Medical School, Minneapolis, Minnesota, USA; Division of Cardiology, Department of Pediatrics, Children's National Hospital, George Washington University School of Medicine, Washington, DC, USA

AARTI S. DALAL, DO
Assistant Professor of Pediatrics, Associate Director of Pediatric Electrophysiology, Division of Cardiology, Monroe Carell Jr

Children's Hospital, Vanderbilt University, Nashville, Tennessee, USA

SOHAM DASGUPTA, MD
Assistant Professor, Division of Pediatric Cardiology, Department of Pediatrics, Norton Children's Hospital, University of Louisville, Louisville, Kentucky, USA

ANNE M. DUBIN, MD, FHRS
Clinical Professor, Chief of Pediatric Cardiology, Lucile Packard Children's Hospital at Stanford University, Palo Alto, California, USA

CAROLINA A. ESCUDERO, MD, MSc
Assistant Professor, University of Alberta, Pediatric Cardiology and Electrophysiology, Stollery Children's Hospital, Edmonton, Alberta, Canada

DAVID GAMBOA, MD
Advocate Children's Heart Institute, Oak Lawn, Illinois, USA

HEATHER M. GIACONE, MD
Clinical Assistant Professor, Department of Pediatric Cardiology, Lucile Packard Children's Hospital, Stanford University, Palo Alto, California, USA

TAYLOR S. HOWARD, MD
Department of Pediatrics, Division of Pediatric Cardiology, Baylor College of Medicine, Texas Children's Hospital, Houston, Texas, USA

PETER P. KARPAWICH, MSc, MD, FAAP, FACC, FAHA, FHRS
Professor, Department of Pediatrics, Central Michigan University College of Medicine, Director, Cardiac Electrophysiology, The Children's Hospital of Michigan, Detroit, Michigan, USA

ROHAN KUMTHEKAR, MD
Division of Cardiology, Nationwide Children's Hospital, Department of Pediatrics, The Ohio State University College of Medicine, Columbus, Ohio, USA

GUILLAUME LECLAIR, MDCM
Pediatric and Congenital Electrophysiology Fellow, Department of Pediatrics, Faculty of Medicine and Dentistry, University of Alberta,

Stollery Children's Hospital, Edmonton, Alberta, Canada

DOUGLAS Y. MAH, MD
Associate Professor, Department of Cardiology, Boston Children's Hospital, Harvard Medical School, Boston, Massachusetts, USA

JEREMY P. MOORE, MD, MS
Professor of Pediatrics, Director of the UCLA Adult Congenital Electrophysiology Program, Division of Cardiology, Department of Medicine, Department of Pediatrics, University of California, Los Angeles (UCLA) Medical Center, Ahmanson/UCLA Adult Congenital Heart Disease Center, UCLA Cardiac Arrhythmia Center, UCLA Health System, David Geffen School of Medicine at UCLA, Los Angeles, California, USA

THOMAS PAUL, MD, FACC, FHRS
Professor of Pediatrics and Pediatric Cardiology, Head, Department of Pediatric Cardiology, Intensive Care Medicine and Neonatology, Georg August University Medical Center, Göttingen, Germany

CHALESE RICHARDSON, MD
Pediatric Cardiology, Zucker School of Medicine at Hofstra/Northwell, The Cohen Children's Heart Center, Northwell Health Physician Partners, New Hyde Park, New York, USA

JEFFREY A. ROBINSON, MD
Assistant Professor, Department of Pediatrics, College of Medicine, University of Nebraska Medical Center, Pediatric Cardiac Electrophysiology, The Criss Heart Center, Children's Hospital and Medical Center, Omaha, Nebraska, USA

MAULLY J. SHAH, MBBS, FACC, FHRS, CCDS, CEPS
Professor of Pediatrics, Director of Cardiac Electrophysiology, The Children's Hospital of Philadelphia, Perelman School of Medicine, University of Pennsylvania, Philadelphia, Pennsylvania, USA; Professor of Pediatrics, Division of Pediatric Cardiology, Children's National Hospital, Division of Cardiology Washington, Washington DC, USA

ELIZABETH D. SHERWIN, MD, FHRS
Associate Professor of Pediatrics, Pediatric
Cardiologist and Electrophysiologist,
Children's National Hospital, Associate
Professor of Pediatrics, George Washington
University School of Medicine & Health
Sciences, Washington, DC, USA

ELIZABETH A. STEPHENSON, MD
Professor of Paediatrics, University of Toronto,
The Hospital for Sick Children, Labatt Family
Heart Centre, Toronto, Ontario, Canada

REINA BIANCA TAN, MD
Assistant Professor, Division of Cardiology,
Department of Pediatrics, NYU Langone

Health and Hassenfeld Children's Hospital,
New York, New York, USA

JEFFREY M. VINOCUR, MD
Department of Pediatrics, Division of Pediatric
Cardiology, Yale School of Medicine, New
Haven, Connecticut, USA

GREGORY WEBSTER, MD, MPH
Division of Cardiology, Ann & Robert H. Lurie
Children's Hospital of Chicago, Northwestern
University Feinberg School of Medicine,
Chicago, Illinois, USA

FRANK J. ZIMMERMAN, MD
Advocate Children's Heart Institute, Oak Lawn,
Illinois, USA

Contents

Surgery for congenital heart disease may compromise atrioventricular (AV) nodal conduction, potentially resulting in postoperative AV block. In the majority of cases, AV nodal function recovers during the early postoperative period and may only require short-term pacing support, typically provided via temporary epicardial wires. Permanent pacing is indicated when the postoperative AV block persists for more than 7 to 10 days due to the risk of mortality if a pacemaker is not implanted. Although there is a subset of patients who may have late recovery of AV nodal function, those with continued postoperative AV block will need lifelong pacing therapy.

Insertable cardiac monitors (ICMs) have been used more frequently and in a wider variety of circumstances in recent years. ICMs are used for symptom-rhythm correlation when patients have potentially arrhythmogenic syncope and for less traditional reasons such as rhythm surveillance in patients with genetic arrhythmia syndromes or other diseases with high arrhythmia risk. ICMs have good diagnostic yield in pediatric patients and in adults with congenital heart disease and have a low rate of complications. Implantation techniques should take patient-specific factors into account to optimize diagnostic yield and minimize risk.

 Video content accompanies this article at http://www.cardiacep.theclinics.com.

Transcatheter leadless pacemakers have benefits in congenital heart disease because they eliminate the risks of lead malfunction, venous occlusions, and pocket complications. This newest pacemaker's utility in this population has been limited by the large sheath and delivery system, need for atrioventricular synchronous pacing, lack of explantation options, and possible lack of adequate access to the sub-pulmonary ventricle. With careful planning, leadless pacing can be successfully performed in these patients. Consideration of nonfemoral access, alternative implant sites to avoid myocardial scar or prosthetic material, anticoagulation for patients with persistent intracardiac shunts or systemic ventricular implantation, and operator experience are critical.

Peter P. Karpawich and Henry Chubb

Heart failure in patients with congenital heart disease (CHD) stems from unique causes compared with the elderly. Patients with CHD face structural abnormalities and malformations present from birth, leading to altered cardiac function and potential complications. In contrast, elderly individuals primarily experience heart failure due to age-related changes and underlying cardiovascular conditions. Cardiac resynchronization therapy (CRT) can benefit patients with CHD, although it presents numerous challenges. The complexities of CHD anatomy and limited access to appropriate venous sites for lead placement make CRT implantation demanding.

Frank J. Zimmerman and David Gamboa

Cardiac resynchronization therapy (CRT) for congenital heart disease has shown promising suucess as an adjunct to medical therapy for heart failure. While cardiac conduction defects and need for ventricular pacing are common in congential heart disease, CRT indications, techniques and long term outcomes have not been well establaished. This is a review of the techniques nad short term outcomes of CRT for the following complex congenital heart disease conditions: single ventricle physiology, systemic right ventricle, and the subpulmonic right ventricle.

Jeremy P. Moore and Aarti S. Dalal

For patients with congenital heart disease (CHD), chronic ventricular pacing may lead to progressive cardiomyopathy owing to electromechanical dyssynchrony. Cardiac conduction system pacing (CSP) has been proposed as a physiologic pacing strategy—directly engaging the His–Purkinje system and preserving electromechanical synchrony. CSP may be indicated for a wide variety of children and adults with CHD and has emerged as an important tool in the armamentarium for cardiac implantable electronic device operators. This review provides the rationale, background, and supportive evidence for CSP in patients with CHD and discusses implant strategies and outcomes in the context of dominant ventricular morphologic categories.

Reina Bianca Tan, Elizabeth A. Stephenson, and Anica Bulic

Epicardial cardiac implantable electronic device implant remains a common option in pediatric patients and certain patients with congenital heart disease due to patient size, complex anatomy, residual intracardiac shunts, and prior surgery precluding transvenous implant. Advantages include the lack of thromboembolic and vascular risks and ability to implant during concomitant surgery. Significant disadvantages include the occurrence of lead dysfunction that can result in bradycardia events in pacemaker patients, inappropriate shocks in implantable cardiac defibrillator patients, and overall a more invasive procedure.

 Video content accompanies this article at http://www.cardiacep.theclinics.com.

Pediatric patients with congenital heart disease present unique challenges when it comes to cardiac implantable electronic devices. Pacing strategy is often determined by patient size/weight and operator experience. Anatomic considerations, including residual shunts, anatomic obstructions and barriers, and abnormalities in the native conduction system, will affect the type of CIED implanted. Given the young age of patients, it is important to have an "eye on the future" when making pacemaker/defibrillator decisions, as one can expect several generator changes, lead revisions, and potential lead extractions during their lifetime.

Risk stratification for sudden death should be discussed with patients with congenital heart disease at each stage of personal and cardiac development. For most patients, risk is low through teenage years and the critical factors to consider are anatomy, ventricular function, and symptoms. By adulthood, these are supplemented by screening for atrial arrhythmias, ventricular arrhythmias, and pulmonary hypertension. Therapies include medication, ablation, and defibrillator placement.

Pediatric and congenital heart disease patients may require cardiac implantable electronic device implantation, inclusive of pacemaker, ICD, and implantable cardiac monitor, for a variety of etiologies. While leads, generators, and monitors have decreased in size over the years, they remain less ideal for the smallest patients. The potential for a miniature pacemaker, fetal micropacemaker, improving leadless technology, and rechargeable devices creates hope that the development of pediatric-focused devices will increase. Further, alternative approaches that avoid the need for a transvenous or surgical approach may add more options to the toolbox for the pediatric and congenital electrophysiologist.

This article reviews various opportunities to translate established and novel tools and techniques used in adult electrophysiology to pediatrics and the adult congenital heart disease population. There is a specific focus on preoperative management of special population, implantation techniques, and postoperative programming of devices.

Pediatric electrophysiologists believe that there is a paucity of pediatric-specific cardiac implantable electronic devices (CIEDs) available for their patients. Specific patient characteristics such as vascular size, intracardiac anatomy, and expected somatic growth limit the types of CIED implants possible for pediatric and congenital heart disease (CHD) patients. These patients demonstrate higher CIED-related complication rates compared with adults. As the number of pediatric and CHD patients who require CIEDs increases, so does the need for advocacy. Fortunately, collaboration among the Food and Drug Administration, industry, and pediatric societies has led to the improvement of regulations and support for clinical trials.

CARDIAC ELECTROPHYSIOLOGY CLINICS

SERIES OF RELATED INTEREST

Cardiology Clinics
https://www.cardiology.theclinics.com/
Interventional Cardiology Clinics
https://www.interventional.theclinics.com/
Heart Failure Clinics
https://www.heartfailure.theclinics.com/

THE CLINICS ARE AVAILABLE ONLINE!
Access your subscription at:
www.theclinics.com

Foreword

Cardiac Implantable Devices in Pediatric and Adult Congenital Heart Disease Patients: Not Just Hocus Pocus!

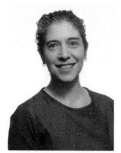 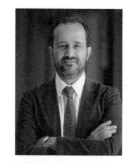

Emily P. Zeitler, MD, MHS, FHRS   Luigi di Biase, MD, MHS, FHRS

Consulting Editors

The old pediatrics saying reminding us that "Children are not just small adults" may not be any truer than when it comes to electrophysiology. As opposed to age-related conduction disease and heart failure, which make up the bulk of adult device implantation scenarios, pediatric patients and those with adult congenital heart disease (ACHD) make up a more diverse group. This diversity presents challenges for the implantation and management of cardiac implantable electronic devices (CIEDs), which, in many cases, need to last an entire lifetime rather than a fraction of one despite the fact that nearly all of the hardware is designed for the latter. Nonetheless, the brilliant, creative, and incredibly skilled group of pediatric electrophysiologists continue to pull rabbits out of hats.

Speaking of magic, Drs Beach and Shah should be applauded for the thoughtful series of topics included in this issue. The issue begins with the most fundamental application of CIEDs in pediatric patients: pacing for postoperative atrioventricular block by Drs Robinson, Leclair, and Escudero. This complication of heart surgery has been the stubborn dark magic that accompanies the lifesaving and highly evolved surgical therapies that have sustained the lives of countless patients born with congenital heart disease. This foundational review then makes way for a journey through the evolution in device-based therapies for pediatric and ACHD patients.

For example, the operators who can achieve cardiac resynchronization therapy in patients with congenital heart disease as described by Drs Zimmerman and Gamboa seem like magicians getting leads to places that do not always seem possible. And, as a potential alternative to traditional cardiac resynchronization therapy, Drs Moore and Dalal review the application of conduction system pacing for patients with congenital heart disease—an example of adult-to-pediatric sleight of hand to apply one of the recent evolutions in adult CIED science to a group that may stand to benefit significantly and may have limited alternative options.

Card Electrophysiol Clin 15 (2023) xiii–xiv
https://doi.org/10.1016/j.ccep.2023.08.002
1877-9182/23/© 2023 Published by Elsevier Inc.

Given the extended period of CIED implantation for pediatric and ACHD patients, lead management figures quite prominently. Drs Dasgupta and Mah provide a roadmap for how the "show must go on" even when there are lead failures or infections. Perhaps emerging tools for delivering CIED care to pediatric and ACHD patients will alleviate some of the problems with lead management or at least put more "tricks up our sleeves," including, for example, leadless pacing, which is reviewed by Drs Sherwin and Shah.

The issue concludes with inspiring reviews; we have much to look forward to in this space. Emerging CIED technologies in pediatric and ACHD patients are reviewed by Drs Clark and Berul, and Drs Giacone and Dubin highlight unmet needs.

We are so pleased to present this issue and are grateful that Drs Beach and Shah chose to cast their benevolent spell over us with this enchanting set of reviews. It is the first time that *Cardiac Electrophysiology Clinics* has covered this topic—and it was about time!

Emily P. Zeitler, MD, MHS, FHRS
Dartmounth-Hitchock Medical Center
1 Medical Center Drive
Lebanon, New Hampshire 03756, USA

Luigi di Biase, MD, MHS, FHRS
Montefiore Medical Center
111 East 210th Street
Bronx, NY 10467, USA

E-mail addresses:
emily.p.zeitler@hitchcock.org (E.P. Zeitler)
dibbia@gmail.com (L. di Biase)

Preface

Advances in Cardiac Implantable Electronic Devices and Congenital Heart Disease

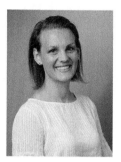
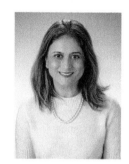

Cheyenne M. Beach, MD, CEPS-P   Maully J. Shah, MBBS, FACC, FHRS, CCDS, CEPS

Editors

Cardiac implantable electronic devices (CIEDs) are a mainstay of treatment for many electrophysiologic diseases. Throughout the last century we have seen remarkable advances in the approaches used for CIED implantation and management. The initial goal of CIED use was to achieve patient stability and survival. As we have learned more about conduction system function and cardiac contractility, parallel advances in technology have allowed us to set our sights on achieving relatively normal physiology and good quality of life for our patients.

CIED use in adult patients is typically well supported with robust science, literature, and guidelines. The same is not true for pediatric and adult congenital heart disease (ACHD) patients due to dramatically smaller numbers of those affected and vast heterogeneity in cardiac anatomy, vascular access, approach to repair or palliation, and resulting physiology. Management approaches must therefore be individualized based on data reported in smaller studies and case series, cautious extrapolation of data from adult patients with structurally normal hearts, expert opinion, innovation, and shared decision making. Collaboration among providers and institutions and with our colleagues in adult electrophysiology is imperative to provide the best care possible for our patients and to advance the field.

In this issue of the *Cardiac Electrophysiology Clinics*, we explore the nuances of device indications, implantation techniques, needs, and future prospects that arise in pediatric and ACHD patients. We kindly thank the expert contributors for their thoughtful illumination of the history and complexity seen in our patients. The issue begins with a description of the use of pacemakers for surgical atrioventricular block, the incidence of which has remained fairly stable despite significant advances in surgical technique. The evolving role of insertable cardiac monitors and the emerging role of leadless pacing are then explored. Next, contributing authors detail indications and techniques for cardiac resynchronization

Card Electrophysiol Clin 15 (2023) xv–xvi
https://doi.org/10.1016/j.ccep.2023.08.001
1877-9182/23/© 2023 Published by Elsevier Inc.

cardiacEP.theclinics.com

therapy and physiologic pacing with particular attention paid to patients with systemic right ventricles (eg, congenitally corrected transposition of the great arteries), subpulmonic right ventricles (eg, tetralogy of Fallot), and single ventricles. Exploration of the benefits, risks, and nontraditional use of epicardial devices is then followed by reviews of lead management and prediction of sudden cardiac death in our patient populations. Finally, we explore emerging technologies in small patients, the translation of tools and techniques from the adult electrophysiology world, and current device needs in these patients. These reviews highlight the paucity of pediatric-specific technology and the importance of collaboration among innovators, the FDA, industry, and both pediatric and adult electrophysiology societies.

We would like to express our gratitude to Drs Zeitler and Prutkin for inviting us to edit this issue of the *Cardiac Electrophysiology Clinics*. It has been an absolute pleasure to work with them and this outstanding group of authors.

Cheyenne M. Beach, MD, CEPS-P
Department of Pediatrics
Section of Pediatric Cardiology
Yale University School of Medicine
333 Cedar Street
New Haven, CT 06520, USA

Maully J. Shah, MBBS, FACC, FHRS, CCDS, CEPS
The Children's Hospital of Philadelphia
Perelman School of Medicine
University of Pennsylvania
3401 Civic Center Boulevard
Philadelphia, PA 19104, USA

E-mail addresses:
cheyenne.beach@yale.edu (C.M. Beach)
shahm@chop.edu (M.J. Shah)

Pacing in Pediatric Patients with Postoperative Atrioventricular Block

Jeffrey A. Robinson, MD[a,b], Guillaume Leclair, MDCM[c,d],
Carolina A. Escudero, MD, MSc[e,f],*

KEYWORDS

- Postoperative • AV block • Atrioventricular • Heart block • Congenital heart disease • Pacemaker

KEY POINTS

- Postoperative atrioventricular (AV) block is relatively common after surgery for congenital heart disease, with many cases resolving in the immediate postoperative period.
- Temporary pacing support is required for postoperative AV block to maintain patient hemodynamics while monitoring for recovery of AV node function.
- Persistent postoperative advanced second- or third-degree AV block lasting greater than 7 to 10 days is an indication for implantation of a permanent pacemaker.
- Some patients may have late recovery of postoperative AV block, whereas those with continued persistent advanced second- or third-degree AV block are managed with lifetime pacing support.

INTRODUCTION

Normal electrical conduction from the atria to the ventricles relies on an intact atrioventricular (AV) node. There are several different etiologies that can cause temporary or permanent compromise to the AV node, which may result in complete heart block and bradycardia (Fig. 1). For patients undergoing heart surgery, postoperative AV block requires significant consideration for clinical management.

Over the last century, the pioneering field of surgery for congenital heart disease (CHD) has been intertwined with growing knowledge of the anatomy, physiology, characteristics, and vulnerabilities of the AV node, especially pertaining to specific congenital heart lesions and surgical techniques. In the earliest era of open-heart surgery for CHD (ventricular septal defect (VSD), tetralogy of Fallot, and complete AV septal defect repairs), persistent postoperative AV block was a fatal complication associated with 100% mortality.[1] Early management was limited to pharmacologic treatment of AV block with short-term medications including isoproterenol.[2] Since then, device technology has made possible both temporary and permanent pacing of the heart to overcome the physiologic consequences of AV block.

With time and increasing experience, modern CHD teams have developed protocols and technologies to treat a wide range of pediatric patients with postoperative AV block. This review herein highlights the current knowledge on.

- Incidence and risk factors for postoperative AV block in pediatric patients with CHD
- Role of temporary postoperative cardiac pacing

[a] Department of Pediatrics, College of Medicine, University of Nebraska Medical Center, Omaha, NE, USA; [b] Pediatric Cardiac Electrophysiology, The Criss Heart Center, Children's Hospital and Medical Center, 8200 Dodge Street, Omaha, NE 68114, USA; [c] Department of Pediatrics, Faculty of Medicine and Dentistry, University of Alberta, Alberta, Canada; [d] Stollery Children's Hospital, 4C1.19 WMC, 8440-112 Street, Edmonton, Alberta T6G 2B7, Canada; [e] University of Alberta, Edmonton, Alberta, Canada; [f] Pediatric Cardiology and Electrophysiology, Stollery Children's Hospital, Edmonton, Alberta, Canada
* Corresponding author. Stollery Children's Hospital, 4C1.19 WMC, 8440-112 Street, Edmonton, Alberta T6G 2B7, Canada.
E-mail address: escudero@ualberta.ca

Card Electrophysiol Clin 15 (2023) 401–411
https://doi.org/10.1016/j.ccep.2023.06.008

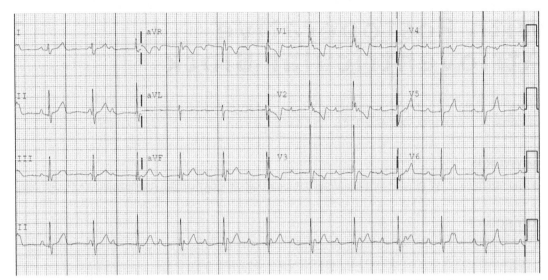

Fig. 1. ECG for an infant with postoperative AV block. Note the complete AV dissociation (seen most clearly in lead II) with regular ventricular rate that is bradycardia for age, which is a typical appearance of postoperative complete heart block.

- Indications for permanent cardiac pacing
- Modes and technology for permanent pacing
- Outcomes and long-term prognosis for pediatric patients with CHD and postoperative AV block

INCIDENCE AND RISK FACTORS

The overall incidence of persistent postoperative AV block is approximately 0.3% to 3% of all pediatric patients undergoing surgery with cardiopulmonary bypass (CPB) for CHD.[3–10] When cases of both transient and persistent postoperative AV block are accounted for, centers have reported up to 6.2% of pediatric CHD patients being affected.[5] In addition, it has been noted that rates of postoperative AV block have not changed significantly over the past several decades for patients with CHD, despite advancements in surgical techniques. Although age itself at the time of surgery has not been found to be an independent risk factor for postoperative AV block, an overall trend for an increased number of surgeries before 24 months of age may be contributing to the continued numbers of patients with postoperative AV block in recent years.[11]

As outlined in **Box 1**, specific CHD lesions have been associated with an increased risk of postoperative AV block, including left ventricular (LV) outflow tract obstruction, L-transposition of the great arteries (L-TGA), and AV septal defects. **Box 1** also outlines particular surgeries for CHD that have been documented to have a higher risk of postoperative AV block including the double-

switch operation, AV valve replacement, and those associated with VSD repair.

For pediatric CHD patients with transient AV block after CPB, Ayyildiz and colleagues reported a median time to resolution of 3 days (range 1–20 days).[5] Here, documented junctional ectopic tachycardia in the postoperative intensive care unit was the only distinguishing factor found in an increased percentage of patients with transient AV block (41%) compared with those diagnosed with permanent postoperative AV block (13%).[5] Weindling and colleagues documented that 63% of pediatric CHD patients with postoperative AV block were transient (resolving by postoperative day [POD] 30), with a resolution of AV block in 42% by POD 2, 81% by POD 7%, and 97% by POD 9.[4] Comparable resolution of transient AV block is reported by the Pediatric Cardiac Critical Care Consortium, with 50% of postoperative patients with CHD recovering AV conduction by POD 2, and 94% by POD 10.[10]

Recurrence of postoperative AV block following initial resolution remains difficult to predict, with up to 9% of patients with initial resolution of transient complete (third-degree) AV block found to subsequently have either documented intermittent or persistent second-degree AV block (Mobitz type I or II) or high-grade second-degree AV block within the first year.[4] Separately, unpredictable development of progressive AV block has been noted with discordant AV connections, AV septal (canal) defects, and heterotaxy syndrome.[9]

Multiple authors have also found that a longer time to resolution of transient complete AV block (patients with a return of AV node conduction at 7 or more days vs those with resolution of AV block within <7 days) is associated with a 13-fold greater risk of recurrent (or late) complete AV block.[11,12] Other predictive factors for late complete AV block have remained elusive.[7,13] Given that almost all patients with transient AV block had resolution by 10 days, emphasis has been given to the implantation of a permanent pacemaker for patients with persistent advanced second- or third-degree AV block at POD 7 to 10, in agreement with indications for device placement per the current consensus statement.[9,11] Currently, it is believed that approximately 1% of all postoperative pediatric patients with CHD require permanent pacemaker placement before hospital discharge.[10,14]

TEMPORARY POSTOPERATIVE PACING

Most pediatric patients with postoperative AV block will regain AV conduction by POD 7 and nearly all will have recovery by POD 10.[4,10] If 1:1 AV conduction is not present, temporary postoperative pacing is used to ensure an adequate ventricular rate and preserve cardiac output. In the case of postoperative AV block, there is improved hemodynamic stability with temporary pacing by

(1) providing appropriate ventricular rate and (2) in the case of dual-chamber pacing, ensuring AV synchrony. This allows for time for observation of AV conduction while awaiting AV node recovery before a decision is made to proceed with a permanent pacing system.

Transcutaneous, transvenous, and epicardial systems are available options to provide temporary pacing; of these, temporary epicardial wires are most common in the postoperative setting and are often implanted at the time of surgery (**Fig. 2**). Although significant advancements have been made in the devices used for temporary postoperative pacing since the 1950s, the overall implantation techniques have been relatively unchanged.

Temporary Epicardial Pacing

Temporary epicardial pacing has been covered by excellent reviews to which we refer the reader.[15,16] The presence of intraoperative arrhythmias and a prolonged aortic cross-clamp time is associated with the therapeutic and diagnostic use of temporary pacing wires.[17] Although practice varies by surgical center, many will place temporary epicardial wires as a standard for patients with CHD associated with a higher risk of dysrhythmias and/or postoperative AV block. The surgical implantation technique allows for easy removal by gentle traction when the wires are no longer needed.

Temporary epicardial wires are available in both unipolar and bipolar configurations. Unipolar systems consist of a cathode attached to the epicardium and an anode in the subcutaneous tissue or associated with a dermal patch. Unipolar systems create a larger pacing spike on the surface electrocardiogram and are less costly than bipolar wires.

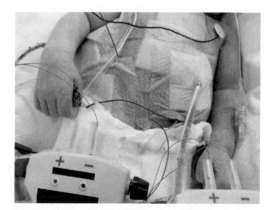

Fig. 2. Temporary postoperative epicardial wire setup. By informal convention, the epicardial wires exiting on the right of the chest are atrial wires (attached to blue connector) and the ventricular wires exit through the left (attached to white connector).

Bipolar wires have both the anode and cathode attached to the epicardial surface and allow for lower capture thresholds compared with unipolar leads. Streamline bipolar leads are available with a coaxial structure that includes optimally spaced discrete electrodes.

By informal convention, temporary atrial wires are attached to the right atrium and brought out to the right of the sternum, whereas temporary ventricular wires attached to the ventricle are brought out to the left of the sternum (see **Fig. 2**). Modern temporary pacemakers typically allow for both single- and dual-chamber pacing. Some temporary pacing systems also allow for biventricular pacing (temporary cardiac stimulator PACE 300: Osypka Medical, Berlin, Germany). Temporary biventricular pacing has been shown to improve cardiac output in patients with CHD, including single ventricle anatomy, with and without postoperative arrhythmias including postoperative AV block.[18–22]

In postoperative AV block, the ideal pacing system should allow for AV synchrony, particularly in cases of CHD where patients are more dependent on the atrial kick for optimal ventricular filling and cardiac output. Temporary pacing follows the same generic code classified by the Heart Rhythm Society and British Pacing and Electrophysiology group.[23] Ideally, pacing should be set to DDD to allow for AV synchrony or alternatively VVI in the presence of poorly functioning atrial wires or a lack thereof (**Fig. 3**). Modern temporary dual-chamber pacemakers allow easy adjustment of pacing mode, lower and upper rate limits, sensitivity, AV delay, post-ventricular atrial refractory period, and both atrial and ventricular outputs. However, the pulse width cannot be modified and the refractory periods and AV delay are not rate-adaptive as they are in permanent pacemakers.

Temporary epicardial leads are not intended for long-term use, and their function will deteriorate over time due to what is thought to be inflammation on the epicardial surface. Their parameters should therefore be checked at least daily in patients dependent on pacing. Both atrial and ventricular pacing thresholds significantly increase after the fourth POD and the P and R wave amplitudes start to deteriorate by the second POD.[24] In addition, unipolar leads are less reliable than bipolar systems.[25,26]

Complications of temporary epicardial pacing seldom occur but can be life-threatening. These include the risk of cardiac tamponade at removal, infection, ventricular arrhythmias, and cardiac perforation.[27–29] Contrary to most modern transvenous permanent pacing systems and some permanent epicardial systems, temporary pacing wires are not considered MRI compatible, even when unconnected. However, patients with retained, short temporary wires have undergone MRI safely.[27]

Troubleshooting Temporary Epicardial Wires in Postoperative Atrioventricular Block

In situations where a dual-chamber bipolar temporary system is poorly functioning due to poor sensing or high capture thresholds, but the patient is not ready or suitable to undergo implantation of a permanent pacing system (eg, if concern for infection or early postoperative status), a few measures can be taken to attempt to maintain AV synchrony using the existing system. Understanding the portion of the system that is acutely malfunctioning is paramount in troubleshooting. Inverting the position of the anode and cathode and therefore inverting the polarity of the wires may provide lower capture thresholds. Converting the system to a unipolar system by anchoring a temporary lead to the subcutaneous tissue or an external dermal patch to serve as the anode may provide better sensing at the cost of likely higher capture thresholds. A high-output asynchronous (VOO) single-chamber pacemaker can be used for very high capture thresholds, but these can cause patient discomfort and local muscle capture. In settings where these options are ineffective, replacing the temporary epicardial wires via sternotomy, transcutaneous pacing, or inserting a temporary transvenous lead or pacing balloon (when the cardiac anatomy and patient size allow) are alternative options. The use of isoproterenol infusions or atropine boluses can temporarily increase the ventricular or junctional escape rates to maintain stability while an alternative short-term or long-term option is established.

Temporary Transcutaneous Pacing

External transcutaneous pacing functions in an asynchronous ventricular (VOO) mode. This setup requires placing the negative adhesive patch on the patient's chest close to the point of maximal impulse and the positive patch on the patient's back directly opposite to the anterior patch. Transcutaneous pacing has many disadvantages for the postoperative patient, including close proximity to the surgical incision site, increased pacing capture thresholds in the presence of pneumothorax or effusions, sedation requirements to maintain a state of unconsciousness due to the extreme discomfort with pacing, and local skin burns. Moreover, this asynchronous system can induce ventricular fibrillation and other dysrhythmias. Rotating the patches every few hours reduces skin trauma. It is recommended to avoid using this pacing method for more than 24 hours.[30]

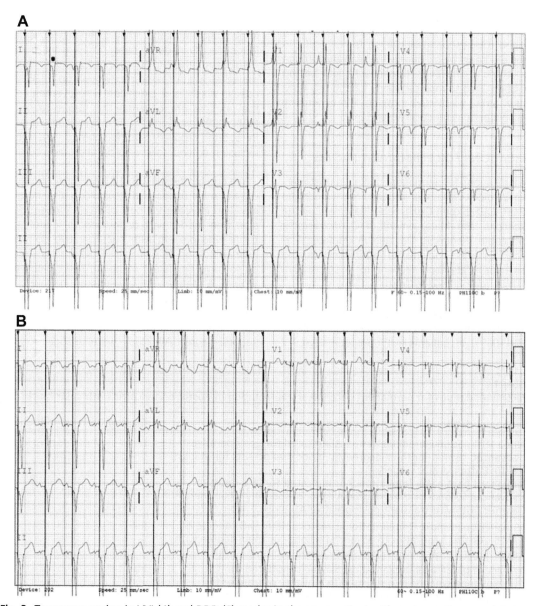

Fig. 3. Temporary pacing in VVI (*A*) and DDD (*B*) modes in the same patient with postoperative complete heart block. Note the VA dissociation in the precordial leads with pacing in VVI mode, which is a characteristic finding of this pacing mode.

Temporary Transvenous Pacing

Temporary transvenous pacing is rarely indicated in pediatric early postoperative AV block, but can be used as a temporizing measure if the patient presents late to a center without the expertise to implant a permanent pacemaker, when the site of future permanent pacemaker implantation is infected or in cases of endocarditis and bacteremia. Temporary pacing can be performed using self-floating balloon-tipped leads or fluoroscopy-guided pacing leads, which both have a risk of acute dislodgement and failure to capture. Temporary transvenous pacing can be established with an actively or passively fixed ventricular lead inserted via the right internal jugular vein, subclavian vein, or femoral vein attached to an externalized implantable single-chamber pacemaker. The use of temporary transvenous pacing with an externalized implantable pacemaker is rarely performed in pediatric patients with postoperative AV block, but is reported in the adult population, with risks of lead malfunction requiring lead repositioning.[9]

Transesophageal Pacing

Isolated transesophageal pacing is not useful in complete heart block due to the inability to pace the ventricle. However, transesophageal pacing has been used to replace poorly functioning temporary atrial wires and provide AV synchrony with epicardial ventricular wires.[20]

INDICATIONS FOR PERMANENT PACING

The indications for permanent pacing in postoperative AV block have been recently reviewed in the 2021 PACES Expert Consensus Statement on the Indications and Management of Cardiovascular Implantable Electronic Devices in Pediatric Patients.[9] Specific indications addressed in the consensus statement relevant to postoperative AV block are outlined in **Table 1**.

The indication for permanent pacemaker implantation after a period of 7 to 10 days stems from natural history data suggesting high mortality (28%–100%) in patients with postoperative AV block who do not undergo permanent pacemaker implantation and the limited benefits of waiting longer for AV node recovery.[4,10,31] In the current surgical era, the 7 to 10 day postoperative waiting period allows AV node recovery in up to 95% of cases, which is a significant improvement over the surgical era covering the 1960s to 1980s (43%–92% recovery).[4,31] The significant variation in reported recovery is attributable to variability in inclusion criteria, follow-up duration, and surgical era.

Waiting for the full 7 to 10 days for AV node recovery may unnecessarily prolong the hospital stay and increase the cost of care. A recent decision tree model was developed to identify patients who present with postoperative complete heart block on POD 0 and POD 4 who will go on to have persistent complete heart block and require a permanent pacemaker implant.[32] In this cohort of 139 patients, 71 (51%) had recovery and 68 (49%) had a permanent pacemaker implanted. Intermittent complete heart block and second-degree AV block were associated with

---

Table 1
Recommendations for permanent pacemaker implantation in postoperative atrioventricular block[9]

Recommendation	Class of Recommendation[a]
Permanent pacemaker implantation is indicated for postoperative advanced second- or third-degree AV block that persists for at least 7–10 d after cardiac surgery. Permanent pacemaker implantation is indicated for late-onset advanced second- or third-degree AV block especially when there is a prior history of transient postoperative AV block.	I
Permanent pacemaker implantation is reasonable for any degree of AV block that progresses to advanced second- or third-degree with exercise in the absence of reversible causes.	IIa
Permanent pacemaker implantation may be considered for unexplained syncope in patients with a history of transient postoperative advanced second- or third-degree AV block. Permanent pacemaker implantation may be considered at <7 postoperative days when advanced second- or third-degree AV block is not expected to resolve due to extensive injury to the cardiac conduction system. Permanent pacemaker implantation may be considered in select patients with transient postoperative advanced second- or third-degree AV block who are predisposed to progressive conduction abnormalities. Permanent pacemaker implantation may be considered for patients with intermittent advanced second- or third-degree AV block not attributable to reversible causes and associated with minimal symptoms that are otherwise unexplained.	IIb

[a] Class I indication: The benefits significantly outweigh the risks and the procedure should be performed. Class IIa: The benefits of the procedure outweigh the risk and it is reasonable to perform the procedure. Class IIb: The benefits outweigh or are equal to the risks and the procedure may be considered or its effectiveness is uncertain.
Modified from Shah MJ, Silka MJ, Silva JNA, et al. 2021 PACES Expert Consensus Statement on the Indications and Management of Cardiovascular Implantable Electronic Devices in Pediatric Patients. Heart Rhythm. 2021;18(11):1888-1924. https://doi.org/10.1016/j.hrthm.2021.07.038; with permission.

recovery (77%). The model suggests that in some cases when patient status and progress allows, it may be reasonable to move forward with permanent pacemaker implant with the presence of persistent complete heart block on POD 4 after LV outflow tract surgery, aortic valve replacement, AV valve replacement, or L-looped ventricles. These principles are similarly reflected in the 2021 consensus statement which indicates that when AV conduction is not expected to resolve in conditions predisposed to conduction anomalies, it may be reasonable to proceed with permanent pacemaker implant before the seventh POD (Class IIb).[9]

MODES OF PERMANENT PACING

After meeting an indication for permanent pacing for postoperative AV block, the type of pacemaker must be selected. The principles and considerations for ventricular pacing in postoperative AV block overlap with those for similar indications, including other causes of acquired AV block and congenital AV block in children and patients with CHD.

Pacing therapy can be provided as single-chamber ventricular pacing, dual-chamber pacing, or biventricular pacing. There are no guidelines to guide the specifics of device selection in the setting of postoperative AV block in children. Dual-chamber pacing is commonly used in postoperative AV block to maintain AV synchrony in the setting of CHD and potential residual hemodynamic lesions. Single chamber ventricular pacing may be selected due to limitations of device size in the case of very small infants, if a low percentage of ventricular pacing is anticipated (such as for infrequent and intermittent AV block), or based on institutional preference. Biventricular pacing may be selected in the presence of existing ventricular dysfunction or concerns for significant worsening of ventricular function in the setting of chronic single-site pacing, such as in the case of L-TGA.[33]

The selection of transvenous or epicardial pacing depends on a variety of factors including patient size and cardiac anatomy, requiring individualized decision-making. Epicardial pacing may be preferred in cases where endocardial access to the ventricle may be challenging or may pose additional risks to the patient, such as small patient size, venous occlusion limiting endocardial access, limitations to ventricular chamber access (eg, Fontan circulation, mechanical tricuspid valve), and intracardiac shunts or single ventricle physiology, which increase the risk of systemic thromboembolism. Transvenous pacing is associated with increased complication rates in young infants but may be an acceptable alternative for pacing in appropriately selected children with postoperative AV block.[34]

When epicardial ventricular pacing is pursued, the selection of an optimal pacing site is of great importance, particularly when a high burden of ventricular pacing is expected. Pacing from the LV apex or lateral LV wall is associated with the greatest likelihood of preserving ventricular function, whereas ventricular pacing from the right ventricular (RV) outflow tract or the RV-free wall is associated with an increased risk of LV dysfunction.[35,36] In transvenous pacing in children, there remains debate regarding the role of RV apical versus RV septal pacing in the preservation of ventricular function.[37] More recently, there is a trend toward increasing pediatric experience and performance of left bundle branch area pacing in children and patients with CHD.[38,39] Further study of the role of endocardial pacing sites and associated ventricular function will be required to optimize outcomes in pediatric transvenous pacing for postoperative AV block.

Although postoperative AV block may be transient, in some cases the placement of "prophylactic" epicardial leads may be performed at the time of the index surgery if there is increased concern for the permanency of the postoperative AV block, such as in patients with L-TGA.[40] This may be performed to avoid an additional sternotomy or thoracotomy in case the AV block is persistent. Leads that have been placed prophylactically at the time of concomitant heart surgery show acceptable survival and pacing characteristics at the time of lead retrieval, necessitating only generator placement at the time of meeting indications for permanent pacing.[40]

OUTCOME AND LONG-TERM PROGNOSIS OF POSTOPERATIVE ATRIOVENTRICULAR BLOCK
Late Resolution of Postoperative Atrioventricular Block

Patients who undergo pacemaker therapy for persistent postoperative AV block may have late resolution of their AV conduction. Batra and colleagues found that 9.7% of patients with postoperative AV block who had a permanent pacemaker implanted had recovery of AV conduction, with recovery occurring by a median of 41 days postoperatively (range 18–113 days).[31] Bruckheimer and colleagues found late resolution of AV conduction in 23% and 21% of patients implanted after greater than 10 and greater than 14 days postoperatively, respectively.[41] Van Geldorp and colleagues demonstrated that in children with postoperative AV block with pacemaker implantation after greater than 14 days postoperatively, there was recovery of AV conduction in 12% with recovery occurring up to 7 years postoperatively.[7] In a contemporary report with similar late resolution of AV block (median 13 days, range 5–117 days), factors associated with increased recovery of AV conduction in a single-center cohort included single ventricle physiology, greater weight, and shorter CPB time.[8] There were no recurrences of complete AV block during follow-up in those who had late recovery of AV nodal function in these studies, which suggests a possible reassuring prognosis and necessitates discussion regarding the need for generator replacement when the generator reaches elective replacement indicator status. Individualized decision-making is required when determining the need for ongoing pacing support for patients with later resolution of AV conduction as extensive data regarding the long-term follow-up for the risk of recurrent AV block in these patients is lacking.

Recurrence of Postoperative Complete Heart Block

Despite relatively early recovery of AV node conduction following pacemaker placement, late complete heart block is known to occur in some patients, with a higher incidence in patients who recovered AV node conduction after POD 7.[12] There is limited evidence that the new occurrence of a bifascicular block (long PR interval with either right bundle branch, left bundle branch, or left axis deviation) after surgery in patients who had transient high grade or complete AV block is at higher risk of a late progression to complete AV block, suggesting that despite recovery there has been damage to the AV node which can progress to complete AV block.[42] Limited data on sudden cardiac death in a subset of 288 patients with repaired tetralogy of Fallot who had transient complete heart block beyond the third POD (8/20) raise concerns regarding the long-term follow-up of patients who do not meet implantation criteria.[43] Therefore, recurrence of second- or third-degree AV block in patients with CHD with no identified reversible cause, particularly with a history of postoperative AV block, is a class I indication for permanent pacemaker implantation.[9]

Complications of Long-Term Pacing

Permanent pacing is necessary for patients with persistent postoperative AV block, but this therapy is associated with potential morbidity over long-term follow-up. Generator depletion and eventual lead failure are expected future sequelae of permanent pacing and require repeated device interventions with associated inherent risks including device infection.[44] Although lead failure occurs in both epicardial and transvenous pacing systems, several studies demonstrate that epicardial pacing is associated with an increased rate of lead complications in children as compared with transvenous pacing, including increased capture threshold requiring intervention and lead fracture.[44,45] Epicardial pacing leads may also predispose children to potential coronary compression.[46] Chronic transvenous pacing in young children is associated with venous occlusion, which has been reported as occurring in 5% to 12% of patients.[44,47,48] Other risks of chronic transvenous pacing include AV valve regurgitation and the risk of requiring transvenous lead extraction over a child's lifetime of transvenous pacing. Individualized decision-making is required when choosing the pacing system to provide these patients with continued pacing support while mitigating their risks of complication as much as possible.

Long-term and high-burden ventricular pacing can be associated with pacing-mediated decreased ventricular function and cardiomyopathy in up to 6% to 13% of pediatric patients.[36,49–51] The association of ventricular pacing and decreased ventricular function in children who may require life-long pacing underscores the importance of selecting pacing sites that are more likely to result in preserved ventricular function.

Injury to the conduction system and subsequent permanent pacing with its potential complications remains a significant problem in congenital heart surgery, particularly in complex biventricular repairs. Methods to avoid the occurrence of complete AV block during surgical repair are of key importance to negate the long-term risks of chronic ventricular pacing. High-density intraoperative mapping of the conduction system, particularly in patients with unpredictable conduction system locations (such as L-looped hearts and heterotaxy syndrome), may enable more precise conduction system localization and mitigate the risk of permanent pacing.[52]

SUMMARY

Postoperative AV block has been reported in up to 6% of pediatric and CHD surgeries. Most of these cases recover AV nodal conduction spontaneously within the first postoperative week, but there remains a risk of recurrent AV block. Patients with postoperative AV block require temporary pacing support to reestablish AV synchrony and maintain cardiac output as the recovery of AV nodal conduction is monitored. The lack of recovery of AV nodal conduction within 7 to 10 days postoperatively is an indication for permanent pacing. Late resolution of postoperative AV block has been reported in up to 23% of patients after pacemaker implantation. Decisions regarding initial pacemaker placement, type of pacemaker, and discontinuation of pacing therapy after late recovery of AV nodal conduction require careful and individualized decision-making to minimize complications while maintaining patient safety.

CLINICS CARE POINTS

- Postoperative atrioventricular (AV) block is commonly encountered after surgery for congenital heart disease.
- Most of the cases of postoperative AV block resolve in the immediate postoperative period, requiring only temporary pacing support to maintain patient hemodynamics while monitoring for recovery of AV node function.
- Persistent postoperative advanced second- or third-degree AV block lasting greater than 7 to 10 days is an indication for implantation of a permanent pacemaker.
- Permanent pacemaker implantation may be considered before 7 to 10 days in a subset of patients with a higher risk of persistent postoperative AV block, including patients after left ventricular outflow tract surgery, aortic valve replacement, AV valve replacement, or L-looped ventricles.
- Late recovery of postoperative AV block can occur in a subset of patients with a low-reported incidence of recurrent AV block.

ACKNOWLEDGMENTS

The authors would like to thank Teresa Hartman, MLS, Education & Research Services Librarian at the University of Nebraska Medical Center for her assistance in conducting the literature searches for this article.

DISCLOSURE

The authors have nothing to disclose.

REFERENCES

1. Lillehei CW, Sellers RD, Bonnabeau RC, et al. Chronic postsurgical complete heart block, with particular reference to prognosis, management, and a new P-wave pacemaker. J Thorac Cardiovasc Surg 1963;46:436–56.

2. Lillehei CW. Discussion of Use of Isuprel in treatment of complete heart block. J Thorac Surg 1957;33:57.

3. Fishberger SB, Rossi AF, Bolivar JM, et al. Congenital cardiac surgery without routine placement of wires for temporary pacing. Cardiol Young 2008; 18(1):96–9.

4. Weindling SN, Saul JP, Gamble WJ, et al. Duration of complete atrioventricular block after congenital heart disease surgery. Am J Cardiol 1998;82(4):525–7.

5. Ayyildiz P, Kasar T, Ozturk E, et al. Evaluation of permanent or transient complete heart block after open heart surgery for congenital heart disease. Pacing Clin Electrophysiol PACE 2016;39(2):160–5.

6. Liberman L, Silver ES, Chai PJ, et al. Incidence and characteristics of heart block after heart surgery in pediatric patients: a multicenter study. J Thorac Cardiovasc Surg 2016;152(1):197–202.

7. van Geldorp IE, Vanagt WY, Vugts G, et al. Late recovery of atrioventricular conduction after postsurgical chronic atrioventricular block is not exceptional. J Thorac Cardiovasc Surg 2013;145(4):1028–32.

8. Madani R, Aronoff E, Posey J, et al. Incidence and recovery of post-surgical heart block in children following cardiac surgery. Cardiol Young 2022;1–7. https://doi.org/10.1017/S1047951122002025.

9. Shah MJ, Silka MJ, Silva JNA, et al. 2021 PACES Expert consensus statement on the indications and management of Cardiovascular implantable Electronic devices in pediatric patients. Heart Rhythm 2021;18(11):1888–924.

10. Romer AJ, Tabbutt S, Etheridge SP, et al. Atrioventricular block after congenital heart surgery: Analysis from the pediatric cardiac Critical care Consortium. J Thorac Cardiovasc Surg 2019;157(3):1168–77.e2.

11. Anderson JB, Czosek RJ, Knilans TK, et al. Postoperative heart block in children with common forms of congenital heart disease: results from the KID Database. J Cardiovasc Electrophysiol 2012;23(12):1349–54.

12. Aziz PF, Serwer GA, Bradley DJ, et al. Pattern of recovery for transient complete heart block after open heart surgery for congenital heart disease: duration alone predicts risk of late complete heart block. Pediatr Cardiol 2013;34(4):999–1005.

13. Nishimura RA, Callahan MJ, Holmes DRJ, et al. Transient atrioventricular block after open-heart surgery for congenital heart disease. Am J Cardiol 1984; 53(1):198–201.

14. Lin A, Mahle WT, Frias PA, et al. Early and delayed atrioventricular conduction block after routine surgery for congenital heart disease. J Thorac Cardiovasc Surg 2010;140(1):158–60.

15. Batra A, Balaji S. Post operative temporary epicardial pacing: when, how and why? Ann Pediatr Cardiol 2008;1(2):120.

16. Reade MC. Temporary epicardial pacing after cardiac surgery: a practical review .: Part 1: General

considerations in the management of epicardial pacing. Anaesthesia 2007;62(3):264–71.

17. Bacha EA, Zimmerman FJ, Mor-Avi V, et al. Ventricular resynchronization by multisite pacing improves Myocardial performance in the postoperative single-ventricle patient. Ann Thorac Surg 2004; 78(5):1678–83.

18. Havalad V, Cabreriza SE, Cheung EW, et al. Optimized multisite ventricular pacing in postoperative single-ventricle patients. Pediatr Cardiol 2014; 35(7):1213–9.

19. Pham PP, Balaji S, Shen I, et al. Impact of conventional versus biventricular pacing on hemodynamics and tissue Doppler Imaging Indexes of resynchronization postoperatively in children with congenital heart disease. J Am Coll Cardiol 2005;46(12): 2284–9.

20. Janousek J, Vojtovic P, Chaloupecky V, et al. Hemodynamically optimized temporary cardiac pacing after surgery for congenital heart defects. Pacing Clin Electrophysiol 2000;23(8):1250–9.

21. Zimmerman FJ, Starr JP, Koenig PR, et al. Acute hemodynamic benefit of multisite ventricular pacing after congenital heart surgery. Ann Thorac Surg 2003; 75(6):1775–80.

22. Elmi F, Tullo NG, Khalighi K. Natural history and Predictors of temporary epicardial pacemaker wire function in patients after open heart surgery. Cardiology 2002;98(4):175–80.

23. Bernstein AD, Daubert JC, Fletcher RD, et al. The Revised NASPE/BPEG generic code for Antibradycardia, adaptive-rate, and multisite pacing. Pacing Clin Electrophysiol 2002;25(2):260–4.

24. Wirtz St, Schulte H, Winter J, et al. Reliability of different temporary Myocardial pacing leads. Thorac Cardiovasc Surg 1989;37(03):163–8.

25. Yiu P. Improved reliability of post-operative ventricular pacing by use of bipolar temporary pacing leads. Cardiovasc Surg 2001;9(4):391–5.

26. Nido PD, Goldman BS. Temporary epicardial pacing after open heart surgery: complications and Prevention. J Card Surg 1989;4(1):99–103.

27. Gupta P, Jines P, Gossett JM, et al. Predictors for use of temporary epicardial pacing wires after pediatric cardiac surgery. J Thorac Cardiovasc Surg 2012;144(3):557–62.

28. Carroll KC, Reeves LM, Andersen G, et al. Risks associated with removal of ventricular epicardial pacing wires after cardiac surgery. Am J Crit Care 1998;7(6):444–9.

29. Chun KJ, Gwag HB, Hwang JK, et al. Is transjugular insertion of a temporary pacemaker a safe and effective approach? Widmer J. PLoS One 2020; 15(5):e0233129.

30. Batra AS, Zeltser I. Temporary pacing in children. In: Shah M, Rhodes L, Kaltman J, editors. Cardiac pacing and Defibrillation in pediatric and congenital heart disease. Incorporated: John Wiley & Sons; 2017. p. 198.

31. Batra AS, Wells WJ, Hinoki KW, et al. Late recovery of atrioventricular conduction after pacemaker implantation for complete heart associated with surgery for congenital heart disease. J Thorac Cardiovasc Surg 2003;125(6):1291–3.

32. Duong SQ, Shi Y, Giacone H, et al. Criteria for early pacemaker implantation in patients with postoperative heart block after congenital heart surgery. Circ Arrhythm Electrophysiol 2022;15(11):e011145.

33. Hofferberth SC, Alexander ME, Mah DY, et al. Impact of pacing on systemic ventricular function in L-transposition of the great arteries. J Thorac Cardiovasc Surg 2016;151(1):131–8.

34. Vos LM, Kammeraad JAE, Freund MW, et al. Long-term outcome of transvenous pacemaker implantation in infants: a retrospective cohort study. Europace 2016. euw031. doi:10.1093/europace/euw031.

35. Siddharth CB, Relan J. Is left ventricular superior to right ventricular pacing in children with congenital or postoperative complete heart block? Interact Cardiovasc Thorac Surg 2021;33(1):131–5.

36. Janoušek J, van Geldorp IE, Krupičková S, et al. Permanent cardiac pacing in children: choosing the optimal pacing site: a multicenter study. Circulation 2013;127(5):613–23.

37. Silvetti MS, Ammirati A, Palmieri R, et al. What endocardial right ventricular pacing site shows better contractility and synchrony in children and adolescents? Pacing Clin Electrophysiol PACE 2017; 40(9):995–1003.

38. Li J, Jiang H, Cui J, et al. Comparison of ventricular synchrony in children with left bundle branch area pacing and right ventricular septal pacing. Cardiol Young 2023;1–9. https://doi.org/10.1017/S1047951122003675.

39. Gordon A, Jimenez E, Cortez D. Conduction system pacing in pediatrics and congenital heart disease, a single center Series of 24 patients. Pediatr Cardiol 2022. https://doi.org/10.1007/s00246-022-02942-9.

40. Cohen MI, Rhodes LA, Spray TL, et al. Efficacy of prophylactic epicardial pacing leads in children and young adults. Ann Thorac Surg 2004;78(1): 197–202.

41. Bruckheimer E, Berul CI, Kopf GS, et al. Late recovery of surgically-induced atrioventricular block in patients with congenital heart disease. J Interv Card Electrophysiol Int J Arrhythm Pacing 2002;6(2):191–5.

42. Villain E, Ouarda F, Beyler C, et al. [Predictive factors for late complete atrio-ventricular block after surgical treatment for congenital cardiopathy]. Arch Mal Coeur Vaiss 2003;96(5):495–8.

43. Hokanson JS, Moller JH. Significance of early transient complete heart block as a predictor of sudden death late after operative correction of tetralogy of fallot. Am J Cardiol 2001;87(11):1271–7.

44. Wilhelm BJ, Thöne M, El-Scheich T, et al. Complications and risk Assessment of 25 Years in pediatric pacing. Ann Thorac Surg 2015;100(1):147–53.

45. Silvetti MS, Drago F, Di Carlo D, et al. Cardiac pacing in paediatric patients with congenital heart defects: transvenous or epicardial? Eur Eur Pacing Arrhythm Card Electrophysiol J Work Groups Card Pacing Arrhythm Card Cell Electrophysiol Eur Soc Cardiol 2013;15(9):1280–6.

46. Mah DY, Prakash A, Porras D, et al. Coronary artery compression from epicardial leads: more common than we think. Heart Rhythm 2018;15(10):1439–47.

47. Welisch E, Cherlet E, Crespo-Martinez E, et al. A single institution experience with pacemaker implantation in a pediatric population over 25 years. Pacing Clin Electrophysiol PACE 2010;33(9): 1112–8.

48. Bar-Cohen Y, Berul CI, Alexander ME, et al. Age, size, and lead factors alone do not predict venous obstruction in children and young adults with transvenous lead systems. J Cardiovasc Electrophysiol 2006;17(7):754–9.

49. Moak JP, Hasbani K, Ramwell C, et al. Dilated cardiomyopathy following right ventricular pacing for AV block in young patients: resolution after Upgrading to biventricular pacing systems. J Cardiovasc Electrophysiol 2006;17(10):1068–71.

50. Kim JJ, Friedman RA, Eidem BW, et al. Ventricular function and long-term pacing in children with congenital complete atrioventricular block. J Cardiovasc Electrophysiol 2007;18(4):373–7.

51. Gebauer RA, Tomek V, Salameh A, et al. Predictors of left ventricular remodelling and failure in right ventricular pacing in the young. Eur Heart J 2009;30(9): 1097–104.

52. Feins EN, O'Leary ET, Davee J, et al. Conduction mapping during complex congenital heart surgery: Creating a predictive model of conduction anatomy. J Thorac Cardiovasc Surg 2023;165(5):1618–28.

53. Siehr SL, Hanley FL, Reddy VM, et al. Incidence and risk factors of complete atrioventricular block after operative ventricular septal defect repair. Congenit Heart Dis 2014;9(3):211–5.

54. Kasar T, Ayyildiz P, Tunca Sahin G, et al. Rhythm disturbances and treatment strategies in children with congenitally corrected transposition of the great arteries. Congenit Heart Dis 2018;13(3):450–7.

55. Mah DY, Alexander ME, Banka P, et al. The role of cardiac resynchronization therapy for arterial switch operations complicated by complete heart block. Ann Thorac Surg 2013;96(3):904–9.

The Evolving Role of Insertable Cardiac Monitors in Patients with Congenital Heart Disease

Cheyenne M. Beach, MD[a],*, Chalese Richardson, MD[b],
Thomas Paul, MD, FHRS[c]

KEYWORDS

• Insertable cardiac monitor • Congenital heart disease • Syncope • Arrhythmia

KEY POINTS

• In pediatric patients and in those with congenital heart disease, use of insertable cardiac monitors (ICMs) has good diagnostic yield and a low complication rate.
• ICMs should not be used in patients who meet the criteria for implantation of a pacemaker or defibrillator.
• Adult patients with Fontan palliation may particularly benefit from ICM use because they are at a relatively high risk for arrhythmias and may have a higher threshold than others for pacemaker or defibrillator implantation.
• ICMs may be useful for rhythm surveillance in symptomatic and asymptomatic patients who are at high risk for significant arrhythmias.
• ICMs can be inserted in various locations (parasternal, axillary) and orientations, and implantation techniques should take patient-specific factors into consideration.

BACKGROUND

Insertable cardiac monitors (ICMs) are small implantable electronic devices placed subcutaneously for long-term remote monitoring of cardiac rhythm. ICMs were first studied in 1995, with prototypes introduced a few years later. These devices have been shown to be useful for their initial purpose of documenting patients' heart rhythm during episodes of symptoms/syncope, with diagnostic findings in most patients.[1,2] Since their introduction, however, changes in these monitors have led to more widespread use. Early models had battery lives of 15 to 18 months and

required patients to use an external activator to store information. Subsequent generations harbor longer battery lives, now up to 4.5 years, and are approximately one-tenth the size of the first models used. Insertion now requires an incision of less than 1 cm. Events can be patient reported as a "symptom" using an external activator or a phone application or they can be automatically detected using preprogrammed criteria, which can be adjusted remotely in some models.

As for most cardiac devices, ICMs were first studied and used in adult patients. In the early 2000s the first reports of their use in pediatric patients were published.[3] Benefits for pediatric

[a] Section of Pediatric Cardiology, Yale University School of Medicine, 333 Cedar Street, New Haven, CT 06520, USA; [b] Zucker School of Medicine at Hofstra, The Cohen Children's Heart Center, Northwell Health Physician Partners, 1111 Marcus Avenue, Suite M15, New Hyde Park, NY 11042, USA; [c] Department of Pediatric Cardiology, Intensive Care Medicine and Neonatology, Georg August University Medical Center, Robert-Koch-Str. 40, Göttingen D-37075, Germany
* Corresponding author. Section of Pediatric Cardiology, Yale University School of Medicine, 333 Cedar Street, New Haven, CT 06520.
E-mail address: cheyenne.beach@yale.edu

Card Electrophysiol Clin 15 (2023) 413–420
https://doi.org/10.1016/j.ccep.2023.06.001

patients were comparable to those for adults, with good rhythm documentation.[4–7] Adverse events associated with ICM use in pediatric patients were uncommon and manageable and included infection, erosion, skin tenting, and discomfort.[4,7,8] Pediatric patients and adults with congenital heart disease (CHD) have benefited from device modifications, and indications for their use in this patient population are growing.

GUIDELINES FOR INSERTABLE CARDIAC MONITOR USE

In 2009 the European Heart Rhythm Association published a position paper regarding indications for the use of diagnostic implantable and external electrocardiographic (ECG) loop recorders.[9] Key points regarding ICM use included (1) ICMs should only be used when a clinical evaluation is unrevealing; (2) ICMs should not be used in patients with a clear indication for pacemaker, implantable cardioverter-defibrillator (ICD), or other treatment; (3) pretest probability of positive findings should be considered; and (4) the goal of ICM monitoring should be establishing a correlation between ECG findings and symptoms/syncope.[9]

In 2017 the International Society for Holter and Noninvasive Electrocardiology and the Heart Rhythm Society published an expert consensus statement on ambulatory ECG and external cardiac monitoring/telemetry.[10] The investigators noted that appropriate patient selection should consider the diagnostic utility of the monitor in each patient with special reference to cost-effectiveness, the probability of a life-threatening arrhythmia, patient acceptance, local availability and experience, and symptom frequency.[10]

Guidelines for the diagnosis and management of syncope were subsequently published by the European Society of Cardiology in 2018. As had been widely adopted, ICM use was thought to be indicated in the evaluation of patients with recurrent syncope in the absence of high-risk criteria and a high likelihood of recurrence within the battery life of the device. Specific patient cohorts such as those with hypertrophic cardiomyopathy, arrhythmogenic cardiomyopathy, long QT syndrome, and Brugada syndrome were included; ICM consideration was suggested for patients with these diseases and with syncope who were thought to be at overall low risk for sudden cardiac death.[11]

The expanded use of ICMs was discussed in the 2021 expert consensus statement published by the Pediatric and Congenital Electrophysiology Society in collaboration with multiple international heart rhythm and cardiology societies.[12]

Indications for ICM use in pediatric patients with syncope were similar to those noted earlier in adults. ICM use in patients with severe but infrequent palpitations or other symptoms suspected to be due to an arrhythmia was included, as was its use for detection of subclinical arrhythmias in patients with cardiac channelopathies or other diseases associated with significant rhythm abnormalities. Specific recommendations from this document are shown in **Fig. 1**.

INSERTABLE CARDIAC MONITOR USE IN PEDIATRIC PATIENTS

As of September 2022, the LINQ II (Medtronic, Inc., Minneapolis, MN, USA) ICM has received 510(k) clearance from the US Food and Drug Administration for use in pediatric patients older than 2 years with heart rhythm abnormalities requiring long-term monitoring.[13] ICMs have been implanted safely in children younger than two years, however, without report of serious complications. ICMs are now routinely used in pediatric patients for the evaluation of infrequent but severe symptoms like syncope, palpitations, or other symptoms thought to likely be due to an arrhythmia after unrevealing noninvasive cardiac rhythm monitoring. Along with Holter monitoring, external loop recorders, and remote telemetry, ICMs have been reported to provide a diagnostic yield in 43% to 60% of patients at 2 years and in up to 80% of patients at 4 years in the pediatric population.[4,7,14–18]

With increased battery longevity in recent models, a diagnosis related to symptoms can now be established in the great majority of patients undergoing ICM insertion. In some instances, wearable monitors such as an Apple Watch (Apple, Inc., Cupertino, CA, USA) or Kardia (AliveCor, Inc., Mountain View, CA, USA) monitor can be used for rhythm documentation during symptoms, although they require patients to be conscious and able to use the monitor. These devices also require that the monitors be located near enough to patients when events are occurring. Up to now, these devices are only marketed for use in adult patients and frequently need to be purchased by patients.

IMPLANTABLE USE IN PEDIATRIC AND ADULT PATIENTS WITH CONGENITAL HEART DISEASE

The use of ICMs in pediatric and adult patients with CHD has been well described. ICMs are routinely used for diagnostic purposes in patients with severe symptoms that have not been captured by noninvasive monitoring. ICMs are also being used for identification of less severe

COR	Recommendations	LOE
	Insertable Cardiac Monitors	
I	Noninvasive cardiac rhythm monitoring is indicated in all patients prior to placement of an ICM.	B-NR
I	ICM is indicated in syncopal patients with high-risk criteria when comprehensive evaluation does not define a cause of syncope or lead to a specific treatment, and who do not have conventional indications for a pacemaker or ICD.	B-NR
IIa	ICM is reasonable in the evaluation of patients with recurrent syncope of uncertain origin but not a high risk of SCD.	B-NR
IIa	ICM is reasonable in patients with infrequent symptoms (>30-day intervals) suspected to be due to an arrhythmia, when the initial noninvasive evaluation is nondiagnostic.	C-LD
IIa	ICM implantation is reasonable for guiding the management of patients with cardiac channelopathies or structural heart diseases associated with significant rhythm abnormalities.	C-LD
IIb	ICM may be considered in patients with suspected reflex syncope presenting with frequent or severe syncopal episodes.	C-LD
IIb	ICM may be considered in carefully selected patients with suspected epilepsy in whom anticonvulsive treatment has proven ineffective.	C-LD
IIb	ICM may be considered in patients with severe but infrequent palpitations when other monitoring methods have failed to document an underlying cause.	C-LD
IIb	ICM implantation may be considered for detecting subclinical arrhythmias in patients with cardiac channelopathies or other diseases associated with significant rhythm abnormalities.	C-EO

Fig. 1. Recommendations from the 2021 Pediatric and Congenital Electrophysiology Society (PACES) expert consensus guidelines regarding the use of insertable cardiac monitors in pediatric patients. (*From* Shah MJ, Silka MJ, Avari Silva JN, et al. 2021 PACES Expert Consensus Statement on the Indications and Management of Cardiovascular Implantable Electronic Devices in Pediatric Patients. Heart Rhythm 2021 Nov;18(11):1888-1924; with permission.)

symptoms in patients deemed at high risk for clinically significant arrhythmias or for arrhythmia surveillance in asymptomatic patients at high risk for life-threatening arrhythmias who do not qualify for primary prevention ICDs. Miller and colleagues[19] compared the use and utility of first- and second-generation ICMs in pediatric patients at a single institution and, in this way, described their expanding use as well as evolvement of indications over time. Of a total of 208 patients, 38 (18%) had insertion of a first-generation and 170 (82%) underwent insertion of a second-generation device. The indication for ICM placement was syncope in the majority (71%) of patients receiving a first-generation device and was notably less common (48%) in those receiving a second-generation device. Indications for second-generation device placement included inherited arrhythmia syndrome management (40%), palpitations (19%), and ventricular ectopy (11%). It is of note that these data represented a 5-fold increase in use for patients with inherited arrhythmia syndromes, which will be discussed in more detail in a later section.

Bezzerides and colleagues[7] described the use of ICMs in pediatric patients and in adults with CHD at Boston Children's Hospital from 2014 to 2017. A total of 133 patients with a mean age of 15.7 ± 9.1 years (range 3.6 months to 44.6 years) underwent ICM insertion during this period. Eleven (8%) patients were aged less than 5 years at the time of device placement, whereas 26% of all patients had CHD. Indications included syncope in 44%, a genetic arrhythmia syndrome in 20%, palpitations in 16%, structural disease in 11%, a negative electrophysiology study in 4%, and others in 5%. Of the 34 patients with CHD, 18 (53%) had a diagnostic tracing, with approximately half of these showing a rhythm abnormality. Of the 50 patients undergoing ICM placement for a genetic arrhythmia syndrome, 28 (56%) had a diagnostic tracing, with 12 (43%) of these showing a rhythm abnormality. Diagnoses made by ICM were often clinically important, with nearly one-quarter of patients undergoing pacemaker or ICD implantation following diagnostic transmissions. More recent studies have shown similar results, with overall high efficacy of ICM use in pediatric patients with and without CHD.[18]

INSERTABLE CARDIAC MONITOR USE IN ADULTS WITH CONGENITAL HEART DISEASE

ICMs can be extremely useful in adults with CHD. First, the adult congenital heart disease (ACHD) population is at higher risk for life-threatening arrhythmias than the general population, with rhythm disorders being the leading cause of mortality. Risk stratification based on cardiac lesion, method of repair, and clinical variables has improved identification of patients at high risk for sudden cardiac death resulting in a recommendation for pacemaker or ICD implantation for primary prevention of sudden cardiac death in certain patients.[20–22] These models may be further enhanced based on ICM data such as identification of ventricular arrhythmias and rhythm documentation during symptoms. Pacemaker and ICD implantation is associated with increased risk in this population due to complex anatomy, prior surgical procedures resulting in limited exposure to healthy myocardium, higher number of device-related infections, and presence of other cardiac hardware such as mechanical valves. ICM data can help to clarify the benefits and risks of pacemaker or ICD implantation in this higher-risk population.

Among patients with ACHD, ICMs have most commonly been used in those with lesions and physiology that carry an increased risk for clinically important arrhythmias. In a study of 22 adults with CHD receiving ICMs at the Nationwide Children's Hospital, 32% had Fontan palliation and another 32% had tetralogy of Fallot (TOF).[23] Indications for device placement included syncope in 41%, palpitations in 73%, dizziness in 45%, and prior history of arrhythmia in 72%. CHD complexity was considered simple in 9%, moderate in 50%, and complex in 41% of patients. This distribution, with the greatest percentage of patients having moderate-complexity CHD, was probably due to its high prevalence and those patients having an intermediate risk for significant arrhythmias compared with those with more complex cardiac malformations, who are more likely to have a pacemaker or ICD implanted for primary prevention of sudden cardiac death. In the same study, clinically relevant events were detected in almost half (41%) of the patients during the 4-year study period.[23] Actionable findings included atrial tachyarrhythmias, ventricular tachycardia, and asystolic pauses. Patients with Fontan palliation and TOF were specifically discussed because they constituted the majority of patients in the study. Most

(57%) patients with Fontan palliation had a tachyarrhythmia considered to be a positive diagnostic finding that resulted in cardioversion, electrophysiology study, ICD implantation, or initiation of antiarrhythmic medication (**Fig. 2**). Among the patients with Fontan palliation with clinically actionable events, there was no association with systemic ventricular dysfunction or degree of atrioventricular valve regurgitation that would have predicted those with positive findings. In patients with TOF, on the other hand, no tachyarrhythmias were documented. Only one patient with TOF had a positive diagnostic finding, which was a sinus pause resulting in syncope. Although the number of patients was limited, these data may suggest that ICMs are particularly helpful for decision making in patients with Fontan palliation given the high prevalence of tachyarrhythmias and high rate of actionable findings on ICM recordings, especially when considering the challenges and risks of pacemaker or ICD implantation in this population.

INSERTABLE CARDIAC MONITOR USE IN INHERITED ARRHYTHMIA SYNDROMES

ICM use in patients with inherited arrhythmia syndromes has changed dramatically in recent years. Avari Silva and colleagues[24] addressed outcomes of ICM use in this population. The investigators described 20 patients with known or suspected inherited arrhythmia syndromes who underwent ICM implantation between 2008 and 2015. Of these patients, 9 had catecholaminergic polymorphic ventricular tachycardia (CPVT), 8 had long QT syndrome, 2 had arrhythmogenic right ventricular cardiomyopathy, and 1 had Brugada syndrome. Indications varied, with some patients experiencing symptoms, some suspected to be noncompliant to medication, and some being monitored during activity liberalization. Although few tracings during symptoms yielded actionable data, this information can be important and reassuring because it may allow for continuation of activities, reduction of emotional burden, and

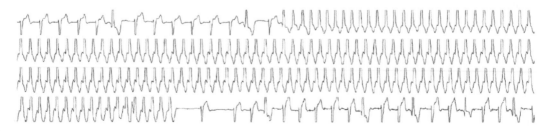

Fig. 2. Documentation of an approximately 60-second episode of monomorphic ventricular tachycardia at 190 bpm associated with syncope in a 52-year-old patient with Fontan palliation and frequent premature ventricular complexes.

improvement of quality of life. Most (81%) automatic transmissions in this study were seen in patients with CPVT, with nearly one-quarter of these requiring further action (**Fig. 3**). These preliminary data suggest that monitoring in select patients with inherited arrhythmia syndromes may be a valuable strategy and will likely be used with increased frequency in the years to come.

INSERTABLE CARDIAC MONITOR PLACEMENT: TECHNICAL ASPECTS

ICMs can be placed using a variety of anesthetic approaches based on patient age, developmental status, and preference as well as patient-specific anesthesia-associated risks. In the study of patients undergoing ICM insertion at Boston Children's Hospital, for example, 50% received conscious sedation, 31% received general anesthesia, and 16% received local anesthesia only.[7] The optimal incision for ICM implantation was initially described as being approximately 2 cm to the left of the sternum in the fourth intercostal space, with the device directed inferolaterally at a 45° angle. An orientation parallel to the sternum has been shown to be noninferior to the diagonal technique and may be a preferred approach in some patients. This orientation may be particularly helpful in small children who may be at increased risk for skin tenting or device erosion with the monitor placed in a traditional diagonal position.[25] Woolman and colleagues compared these parallel and diagonal techniques in 34 patients with a mean age of 12 years (range 1–21 years). Three

patients in each group were younger than 5 years at the time of monitor insertion. Mean R wave amplitudes were similar between groups, and P waves were observed in all cases. One patient with a diagonal approach experienced skin tenting, and no other complications were noted. Although these 2 techniques work well for most patients, size, anatomic, and aesthetic concerns have led to an interest in nonstandardized monitor placement. The position of the heart within the chest should also be considered when inserting an ICM, particularly in patients with CHD. A right-sided implant should be strongly considered in patients with dextrocardia (**Fig. 4**). Bezzerides and colleagues[7] reported that among their cohort of pediatric patients and patients with ACHD undergoing ICM insertion, 64% underwent precordial and 31% underwent axillary placement, while the location was other or not reported in 5%. Although some have found that R wave amplitude was smaller in devices placed via an axillary approach,[7] this location has been found to have similar rates of diagnostic findings[26] and diagnostic yield[7] when compared with precordial placement and may be considered in selected patients (**Fig. 5**). These devices have, however, been found to be associated with more frequent false-positive findings due to noise when compared with those placed in a precordial position.[7] An axillary approach has been chosen due to patient preference and, in some instances, when there has been concern regarding the effect of a precordial device on the quality of cardiac MRI.[26] Axillary ICM placement has been described as vertical

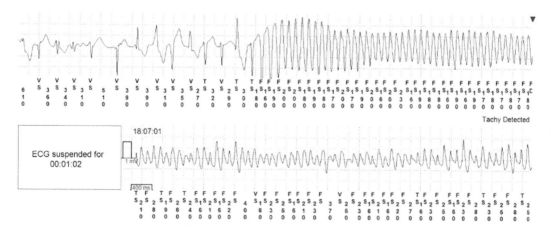

Fig. 3. Documentation of bidirectional ventricular tachycardia with progression to rapid ventricular tachycardia and then ventricular fibrillation in a patient with catecholaminergic polymorphic ventricular tachycardia. The patient experienced syncope followed by spontaneous recovery during this episode, which was documented during an illness associated with vomiting, dehydration, and temporary discontinuation of antiarrhythmic medications due to feeling unwell. Changes in management included improved adherence to medication regimen and observation in a hospital setting during subsequent illnesses precluding the ability to tolerate medications. (*Courtesy of* A. Landstrom, MD, PhD, Durham, NC.)

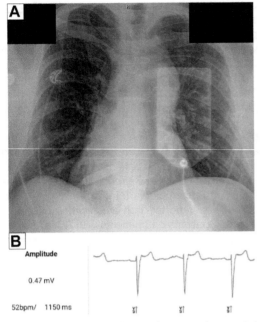

Fig. 4. Right parasternal ICM placement in an adult patient with dextrocardia. (*A*) Chest radiograph showing the location of the ICM. (*B*) High-quality transmission from ICM.

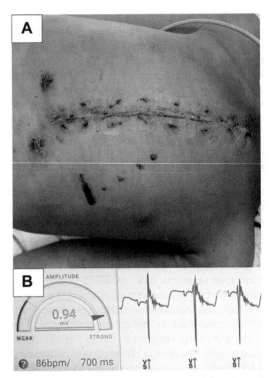

Fig. 6. Placement of an ICM in a 3-year-old patient after recent cardiac surgery. (*A*) The planned location for ICM placement is marked, placing the incision at the inferolateral aspect of the monitor and leaving adequate distance between the medial border of the device and the recent sternotomy incision. (*B*) Excellent amplitude and clear P waves were seen after ICM insertion in the planned location.

along the anterior axillary line, posterior to the lateral edge of the pectoralis major muscle,[26] or as horizontal in the space between the pectoralis major and pectoralis minor muscles.[27] The incision can be made at either end of the planned monitor course based on patient and provider preference. An inframammary approach has been performed by some ICM implanters in girls and young women.[28] Aside from aesthetic concerns, prior and future surgical interventions and complications may also affect optimal device placement (**Fig. 6**).

Although many providers close ICM incisions with sterile adhesive tape or skin glue only, the

use of at least one suture for closure may lead to fewer infections and device erosions.[29] Younger patients may be more likely to manipulate incision sites, increasing these risks; they may also be more active, subjecting the incision to stretch and inadequate approximation in the absence of sutures. In addition, some implanters have found the ICM pocket in younger children to be tighter than in older children, predisposing them to device erosion[30] As a result, in pediatric implantations many operators close ICM incisions with at least one absorbable suture, often followed by sterile adhesive tape or skin glue.

INSERTABLE CARDIAC MONITOR PROGRAMMING

ICMs need to be programmed individually at the time of implantation. Programming parameters are selected based on patient age, indication for device placement, and other patient-specific factors such as activity level and use of antiarrhythmic medications. The goal of ICM programming is to

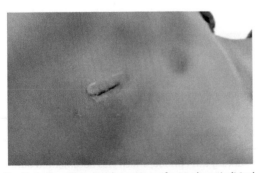

Fig. 5. Left axillary implantation of a Medtronic (Medtronic, Inc., Minneapolis, MN, USA) Reveal XT insertable cardiac monitor in a child. (*Courtesy of* M. Shah, MBBS, Philadelphia, PA.)

maximize the likelihood of receiving clinically important information while minimizing the frequency of false-positive findings, that is, non–patient-activated alerts due to erroneous arrhythmia detection. False-positive findings in pediatric patients and patients with CHD are caused by sinus tachycardia, double counting, T wave oversensing, noise/artifact, signal dropout, and undersensing.[31] Signal dropout and undersensing may be more common in patients with large body habitus and during position changes. Proper identification of false-positive findings and the identification of true-positive findings in the context of frequent false-positive findings require thoughtful programming, manual review of transmissions, knowledge of clinical context, and an understanding of the appearance of each type of false-positive finding. Recently launched AccuRhythm AI algorithms are included in the LINQ II ICM. These algorithms use artificial intelligence to collect data on heart rhythms and significantly reduce the number of false alerts received.[32]

COMPLICATIONS

In the study by Bezzerides and colleagues,[7] 6 patients (4.5%) experienced an ICM-related complication requiring device explantation, including 3 patients with device infection, 2 with device erosion, and 1 with excessive pain. Complications were more frequent in patients younger than 5 years at the time of implantation. Incision closure technique was not described in this study. It may be speculated that particular attention to incision closure in this young population may reduce the risk of complications. Other complications reported in patients undergoing ICM implantation include skin tenting, pneumothorax,[17] and device migration.[33] Importantly, severe complications requiring more than device extraction from its initial location and administration of antibiotics are extraordinarily rare.

SUMMARY

In young patients, ICMs are being used more frequently and for a broader range of indications. Newer-generation devices are much smaller, have longer battery longevity, and are more convenient to use and program than their first-generation counterparts. Various implantation techniques exist and should be chosen based on patient-specific factors as well as patient and provider preference. Diagnostic utility is excellent, and complications are relatively rare in pediatric patients and patients with ACHD, particularly when attention is paid to closure technique.

CLINICS CARE POINTS

- ICMs have increased usage and expanded utility in pediatric patients and in adults with CHD.

- ICMs are useful in patients with inherited arrhythmia syndromes for the detection of symptomatic and subclinical arrhythmias as well as tailoring of antiarrhythmic therapy.

- ICM use in both symptomatic and asymptomatic patients with CHD may aid in the identification of those who would benefit from pacemaker or ICD implantation, recognizing that ICMs should not be used in patients who otherwise meet criteria for these devices.

- Complication rates following ICM insertion are highest in patients younger than 5 years; careful patient selection and consideration of skin closure techniques may reduce risk.

DISCLOSURE

The authors have no commercial or financial conflicts of interest to disclose.

REFERENCES

1. Krahn AD, Klein GJ, Yee R, et al. Final results from a pilot study with an implantable loop recorder to determine the etiology of syncope in patients with negative noninvasive and invasive testing. Am J Cardiol 1998;82(1):117–9.

2. Krahn AD, Klein GJ, Yee R, et al. Use of an extended monitoring strategy in patients with problematic syncope. Reveal Investigators. Circulation 1999;99(3):406–10.

3. Bloemers BLP, Sreeram N. Implantable loop recorders in pediatric practice. J Electrocardiol 2002;35(Suppl):131–5.

4. Babikar A, Hynes B, Ward N, et al. A retrospective study of the clinical experience of the implantable loop recorder in a pediatric setting. Int J Clin Pract 2008;62:1520–5.

5. Frangini PA, Cecchin F, Jordao L, et al. How revealing are insertable loop recorders in pediatrics? Pacing Clin Electrophysiol 2008;31:338–43.

6. Al Dhahri KN, Potts JE, Chiu CC, et al. Are implantable loop recorders useful in detecting arrhythmias in children with unexplained syncope? Pacing Clin Electrophysiol 2009;32:1422–7.

7. Bezzerides VJ, Walsh A, Martuscello M, et al. The real-world utility of the LINQ implantable loop recorder in pediatric and adult congenital heart patients. JACC Clin Electrophysiol 2019;5:245–51.

8. Gass M, Apitz C, Salehi-Gilani S, et al. Use of the implantable loop recorder in children and adolescents. Cardiol Young 2006;16(6):572–8.

9. Brignole M, Vardas P, Hoffman E, et al. Indications for the use of diagnostic implantable and external ECG loop recorders. Europace 2009;11:671–87.

10. Steinberg JS, Varma N, Cygankiewica I, et al. 2017 ISHNE-HRS expert consensus statement on ambulatory ECG and external cardiac monitoring/telemetry. Heart Rhythm 2017;14:e55–96.

11. Brignole M, Moya A, de Lange FJ, et al. 2018 ESC Guidelines for the diagnosis and management of syncope. Eur Heart J 2018;39:669–74.

12. Shah MJ, Silka MJ, Avari Silva JN, et al. 2021 PACES expert consensus statement on the indications and management of cardiovascular implantable electronic devices in pediatric patients. Heart Rhythm 2021;18(11):1888–924.

13. 510(k) Premarket Notification K221962. In: US Food & Drug Administration. 2022. Available at: https://www.accessdata.fda.gov/scripts/cdrh/cfdocs/cfpmn/pmn.cfm?ID=K221962. Accessed May 1, 2023.

14. Moya A, Sutton R, Ammirati F, et al. Guidelines for the diagnosis and management of syncope. Eur Heart J 2009;30:2631–71.

15. Macinnes M, Martin N, Fulton H, et al. Comparison of a smartphone-based ECG recording system with a standard cardiac event monitor in the investigation of palpitations in children. Arch Dis Child 2019; 103:43–7.

16. Pradhan S, Robinson JA, Shivapour J, et al. Ambulatory arrhythmia detection with Zio® XT patch in pediatric patients: a comparison of devices. Pediatr Cardiol 2019;40:921–4.

17. Placidi S, Drago F, Miloni M, et al. Miniaturized Implantable Loop Recorder in Small Patients: an effective approach to the evaluation of subjects at risk for sudden death. Pacing Clin Electrophysiol 2016;39:669–74.

18. Czosek RJ, Zang H, Baskar S, et al. Outcomes of implantable loop monitoring in patients <21 years of age. Am J Cardiol 2021;158:53–8.

19. Miller N, Roelle L, Lorimer D Jr, et al. A single-center experience comparing first- versus second-generation insertable cardiac monitors in pediatric patients. J Innov Card Rhythm Manag 2022;13(6): 5048–56.

20. Oliver JM, Gallego P, Gonzalez AE, et al. Predicting sudden cardiac death in adults with congenital heart disease. Heart 2021;107:67–75.

21. Khairy P, Van Hare GF, Balaji S, et al. PACES/HRS expert consensus statement on the recognition and management of arrhythmias in adult congenital heart disease. Heart Rhythm 2014;11(10):e102–65.

22. Hernández-Madrid A, Paul T, Abrams D, et al. Arrhythmias in congenital heart disease: a position paper of the European Heart Rhythm Association (EHRA), Association for European Paediatric and Congenital Cardiology (AEPC), and the European Society of Cardiology (ESC) working group on grown-up congenital heart disease, endorsed by HRS, PACES, APHRS, and SOLAECE. Europace 2018;20(11):1719–53.

23. Dodeja AK, Thomas C, Daniels CJ, et al. Detection of arrhythmias in adult congenital heart disease patients with LINQ™ implantable loop recorder. Congenit Heart Dis 2019;14(5):745–51.

24. Avari Silva JN, Bromberg BI, Emge FK, et al. Implantable loop recorder monitoring for refining management of children with inherited arrhythmia syndromes. J Am Heart Assoc 2016;5:e003632.

25. Woolman P, Yoon J, Snyder C. Novel technique for cardiac monitor implantation in pediatrics. Pediatr Cardiol 2022;1–5.

26. Anderson H, Dearani J, Qureshi MY, et al. Placement of Reveal LINQ device in the left anterior axillary position. Pediatr Cardiol 2020;41(1):181–5.

27. Miracapillo G, Addonisio L, Breschi M, et al. Left axillary implantation of loop recorder versus the traditional left chest area: a prospective randomized study. Pacing Clin Electrophysiol 2016;39(8):830–6.

28. Kannankeril PJ, Bibeau DA, Fish FA. Feasibility of the inframammary location for insertable loop recorders in young women and girls. Pacing Clin Electrophysiol 2004;27(4):492–4.

29. Gunda S, Reddy YM, Pillarisetti J, et al. Initial real world experience with a novel insertable (Reveal LinQ™@Medtronic) compared to the conventional (Reveal XT™@Medtronic) implantable loop recorder at a tertiary care center – points to ponder. Int J Cardiol 2015;191:58–63.

30. Chaouki AS, Czosek RJ, Spar DS. Missing LINQ: extrusion of a new-generation implantable loop recorder in a child. Cardiol Young 2016;26(7): 1445–7.

31. Afzal MR, Mease J, Koppert T, et al. Incidence of false-positive transmissions during remote rhythm monitoring with implantable loop recorders. Heart Rhythm 2020;17(1):75–80.

32. Ousdigian KT, Cheng YJ, Koehler J, et al. Abstract 14342: artificial intelligence dramatically reduces annual false alerts from insertable cardiac monitors. Circulation 2021;144(1):A14342.

33. Hasnie AA, Hasnie AA, Assaly RA. The case of the migrating loop recorder. J Am Coll Cardiol Case Rep 2019;1(2):156–60.

Leadless Pacemakers in Patients with Congenital Heart Disease

Elizabeth D. Sherwin, MD, FHRS[a], Maully J. Shah, MBBS, FACC, FHRS[b],*

KEYWORDS

- Leadless pacemaker • Pediatric cardiology • Congenital heart disease • Transcatheter pacing

KEY POINTS

- Patients with congenital heart disease (CHD) have an increased need for cardiac pacing due to sinus node dysfunction and atrioventricular block, which may be congenital or postoperative. This population may require decades of pacing with recurrent reoperations and has a higher rate of pacemaker complications.
- CHD presents unique access and anatomic challenges that require preparation and creativity in the use of leadless pacemakers.
- Vascular access, limited options for atrioventricular synchronous pacing, and uncertainty regarding long-term extraction currently hinder the broad use of leadless pacemakers in CHD; further modifications to implant tools and programming options may broaden their utility in these patients.
- Transcatheter leadless pacing can be safe and achievable in select pediatric and adult patients with CHD and can reduce or eliminate the risks of lead malfunction and pocket complications.

 Video content accompanies this article at http://www.cardiacep.theclinics.com.

INTRODUCTION

Transcatheter leadless pacemakers (TLPs) are the latest major innovation in cardiac implantable electronic devices (CIEDs) and have been shown to be a safe and effective option for adults with pacing indications.[1–4] TLPs offer benefits over traditional pacemakers by reducing lead- and pocket-related complications.[1–6]

TLPs may be an alternative for children and patients with congenital heart disease (CHD) for whom repeated sternotomies, thoracotomies, or transvenous systems are unfavorable. However, data in children are limited to case reports and small series.[7–11] Recently, a larger multicenter retrospective Pediatric and Congenital Electrophysiology Society (PACES) registry study showed short-term safety and efficacy of TLP in children comparable to that seen in adults.[12] Although these results are reassuring, there are no guidelines, practice recommendations, or expert consensus statements for the use of these devices in pediatric patients and patients with CHD.

LEADLESS PACING PAST AND PRESENT

TLPs were initially conceptualized in the 1970s. A TLP prototype was first implanted in a dog in 1970 (**Fig. 1**).[13] The device was initially powered by a mercury battery and then an experimental

[a] Division of Pediatric Cardiology, Children's National Hospital, Division of Cardiology Washington, 111 Michigan Avenue, NW, Washington, DC 20010, USA; [b] Cardiac Electrophysiology, The Children's Hospital of Philadelphia, Perelman School of Medicine, University of Pennsylvania, 3401 Civic Center Boulevard, Philadelphia, PA 19104, USA
* Corresponding author. The Cardiac Center, Children's Hospital of Philadelphia, 3401 Civic Center Boulevard, Philadelphia, PA 19104.
E-mail address: SHAHM@chop.edu
Twitter: @MaullyShah (M.J.S.)

Card Electrophysiol Clin 15 (2023) 421–432
https://doi.org/10.1016/j.ccep.2023.06.002

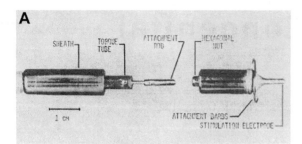

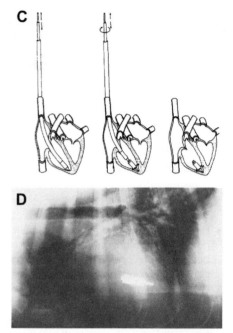

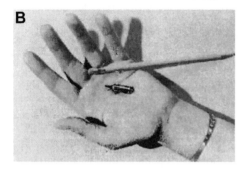

Fig. 1. The first prototype of a self-contained venous catheter-implanted intracardiac pacemaker. (*A*) A capsule-type intracardiac pacemaker with active fixation "attachment barbs" and the triaxial catheter that was used for insertion and attachment. (*B*) The first nuclear-powered intracardiac pacemaker. (*C*) Intracardiac pacemaker insertion sequence. (*D*) Lateral radiograph of intracardiac pacemaker implanted in a dog. (*Adapted from* Spickler JW, Rasor NS, Kezdi P, et al. Totally self-contained intracardiac pacemaker. J Electrocardiol 1970;3(3–4):325–31;with permission.)

beta voltaic nuclear battery. Owing to practical limitations of prior battery technology, commercialization was not implemented. Advances in battery and communication technology allowed for the first in-human implantation of a leadless pacemaker (LP) in 2013 Nanostim (Nanostim Inc, Sunnyvale, CA, USA). This device never received US Food and Drug Administration (FDA) approval and was removed from the market because of premature battery depletion and reports of spontaneous separation of the docking/retrieval button during the LEADLESS II clinical trials.[14,15] The first TLP to receive FDA approval was the Micra VR Transcatheter Pacing System (Medtronic, Minneapolis, MN, USA) in April 2016. This device has been implanted around the world in more than 150,000 adults. A second-generation device (Micra AV) was approved for use in January 2020 and offers a novel sensing mechanism allowing sequential atrial mechanical sensing and ventricular pacing. In May 2023, the FDA granted approval of Micra AV2 and Micra VR2, which have 40% more battery life compared with previous generations.[16]

After cessation of Nanostim LP implantations in 2016, the next TLP under the new ownership of Abbott Medical (Sylmar, CA, USA) was the Aveir VR single-chamber (Abbott Medical, Sylmar, CA)

LP, which received FDA approval in March 2022 based on results of the LEADLESS II phase 2 trial.[15]

TYPES OF FOOD AND DRUG ADMINISTRATION-APPROVED LEADLESS PACEMAKERS

Micra VR (**Fig. 2**): The Micra device is a self-contained, hermetically enclosed, miniaturized single-chamber pacemaker (**Table 1**). This device is implanted in the right ventricle (RV) via a 23F delivery catheter that goes through a 105-cm-long introducer sheath designed for a femoral venous approach.[1,2] The device is fixated via 4 electrically inactive extendable/retractable nitinol tines on the distal end of the device (see **Fig. 2**). The functionality and features of the device are similar to existing single-chamber pacemakers. By design, the device is MRI conditional; its pacing electrodes are situated directly on the capsule, with the cathode located at the tip and the anode located on a ring on the capsule body. The device requires deployment before initial electrical readings; it uses a 3-axis accelerometer for rate responsiveness and offers multiple pacing modes (VVI, VVIR, VOO, OVO). The device can be programmed to "OFF/OOO mode," and when the battery voltage reaches the end of

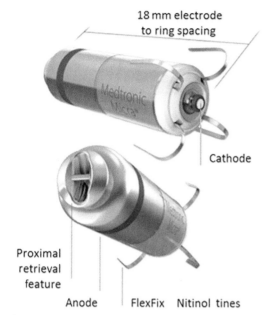

18 mm electrode to ring spacing

Cathode

Proximal retrieval feature

Anode   FlexFix   Nitinol tines

Fig. 2. Micra TPS system components. (Images used with permission from Medtronic, plc © 2023.)

service (EOS) condition it automatically switches to this mode. The Micra does not have a long-term extraction mechanism; at battery depletion, a new device may be implanted alongside it.

Micra AV: Although the characteristics and specifications of the Micra AV are similar to those of the Micra VR, the Micra AV also contains an accelerometer that senses atrioventricular (AV) mechanical activity; it can facilitate AV synchrony by discriminating between the start and end of ventricular systole (A1

and A2, respectively) and localizing the duration of passive and active ventricular filling from atrial activity (A3 and A4, respectively, **Fig. 3**). This device offers VDD, VDI, and ODO pacing modes. The VDD algorithm involves accelerometer signal filtering, automatic threshold adjustments, and switching out of VDD mode during periods of AV conduction and high-sensed patient activity.[17] A limitation of the device is that, irrespective of optimization, AV synchrony correlates inversely with intrinsic sinus rate during predominantly paced periods, with loss of AV synchrony at heart rates greater than 115 bpm.[18] In addition, compared with supine body position, standing and walking have a negative effect on accelerometer signal quality.[18] Therefore, more sedentary patients with lower heart rates may be better candidates for leadless VDD pacing using this device.

Micra VR2 and Micra AV2: The new generation of Micra devices offers approximately 40% longer battery life compared with previous generations. The updated Micra AV2 and Micra VR2 delivery system cup is thicker with a rounded edge to reduce tissue pressure during implantation. The Micra AV2 also includes advanced algorithms for improving AV synchrony and achieving a higher available tracking capability for faster heart rates (increased upper limit from 115 to 135 bpm).[19]

Aveir VR (**Fig. 4**): The redesigned LP (Aveir, Abbott) uses standard transvenous pacemaker battery chemistry (lithium carbon monofluoride) with a 12% longer battery life, an altered form factor (10% shorter, 1.5F wider, 19.5F), a modified docking button enabling retrievability, a specific integrated circuit chip designed to provide an

Table 1
Characteristics of commercially available leadless pacemakers

	Micra VR	Micra AV	Aveir VR
Mass (g)	2	2	2.4
Volume (mL)	0.8	0.8	1.1
Length (mm)	25.9	25.9	38
Outer diameter (O.D.) (mm)	6.7	6.7	6.5
Fixation type	Passive	Passive	Active
Fixation mechanism	Tines	Tines	Nonretractable helix
Electrode spacing (mm)	18	18	24
Steroid elution	Yes	Yes	Yes
Sensor	Accelerometer	Accelerometer	Temperature
Battery longevity	10 y 1.5 v@0.25 ms	10 y 1.5@0.25 ms	10.4 y 2.5 v @0.4 ms
Introducer sheath O.D.	27F	27F	27F
Delivery catheter size	23F	23F	25F

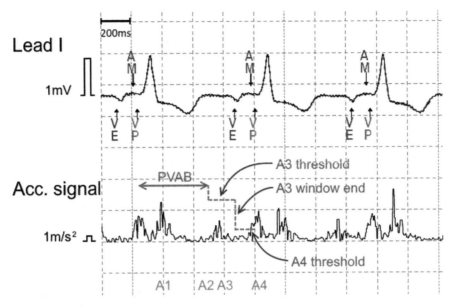

Signal or marker	Occurrence	Function/meaning
A1 signal	After the beginning of the ventricular systole (after the beginning of the QRS complex)	Closure of mitral and tricuspid valve
A2 signal	At the end of the ventricular systole (at the end of the T-wave)	Closure of aortic and pulmonary valve
A3 signal	During ventricular diastole (after the T-wave).	Corresponds to the passive ventricular filling phase (i.e. the E-wave in the TTE)
A4 signal	During atrial systole (after the p-wave).	Corresponds to the active ventricular filling phase (i.e. the A-wave in the TTE)
A7 signal	During fusion of the A3 and A4 signal (i.e. E- and A-wave) due to higher heart rates or lack of AV synchrony	Corresponds to a ventricular filling phase (E/A-fusion in the TTE)
AM	If a mechanical event is sensed during the A3/A4 window above the A3/A4 threshold. Does not occur in VVI+ mode.	Presumed atrial mechanical contraction (A4 signal/A-wave)
AR	If an atrial signal is detected during the PVARP	Atrial refractory event
VE	At the end of the A3 window. Does not occur in VVI+ mode.	Marks the A3 window end according to the PM, is not a physiologic event
VP	If ventricular pacing is delivered	Ventricular pacing
VS	If a ventricular sensed event occurs	Ventricular sensing

Fig. 3. Schematic illustration and explanation of the key atrial sensing parameters. (*Top signal*) The electrocardiogram. (*Bottom signal*) The rectified accelerometer signal that is used to detect the atrial mechanical activity (A4 signal). The PVAB begins once the ventricular pacing stimulus is delivered. At its end, the A3 window starts; it features an A3 threshold to blind the pacemaker for A2 and A3 signals. When the A3 window ends, the "VE" signal is triggered and the A4 window begins. The A4 threshold allows programming an appropriate sensitivity to detect A4. Once a signal is detected either in the A3 window above the A3 threshold or in the A4 window above the A4 threshold it is labeled "AM." After the sensed AV delay, the pacing stimulus is delivered. Adjustment of the atrial sensing parameters (*orange*) is critical for reliable detection of the atrial contraction. AM, atrial mechanical marker; AV, atrioventricular; PM, pacemaker; PVAB, postventricular atrial blanking; PVARP, postventricular atrial refractory period; VE, ventricular end marker. (*From* Neugebauer F, Noti F, van Gool S, Roten L, Baldinger SH, Seiler J, Madaffari A, Servatius H, Ryser A, Tanner H, Reichlin T, Haeberlin A. Leadless atrioventricular synchronous pacing in an outpatient setting: Early lessons learned on factors affecting atrioventricular synchrony. Heart Rhythm. 2022 May;19(5):748-756; with permission.)

expandable platform (to later support a dual-chamber pacing system once approved), and a modified delivery system with a delivery catheter in two length options (30 cm, 50 cm).[15] The device attaches to the RV myocardium with a nonretractable helix to a depth of 1.63 mm. The device's distal end has a double-helix mechanism with an inert outer helix used for mechanical contact with the myocardium and an electrically active inner helix that serves as the cathode.[20] The exposed cathode allows for contact mapping of sensing and pacing thresholds before fixation.

TRANSCATHETER LEADLESS PACEMAKER IMPLANTATION PROCEDURE

Both Micra and Aveir devices are attached to a steerable catheter delivery system designed to

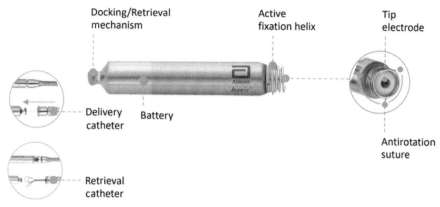

Fig. 4. Components of the Aveir VR pacemaker. (Abbott, Abbott 'A', and Aveir are trademarks of Abbott or its related companies. Reproduced with permission of Abbott, © 2023. All rights reserved.)

be inserted through a femoral vein with the use of an introducer sheath and advanced through the tricuspid valve (TV) into the RV under fluoroscopy, and the device is affixed to the myocardium. The system is fully retrievable and repositionable while the device remains connected to the delivery system. Radiographic contrast is injected using right axial oblique and left axial oblique fluoroscopic projections to determine optimal device positioning (**Fig. 5**A, B, Videos 1 and 2). After electrical threshold testing and determination of stability, the device is released from the delivery system (**Fig. 5**C, D, Videos 3 and 4), after which the delivery catheter and introducer are removed (Videos 5 and 6). The vascular access site is typically closed with a subcutaneous "figure-of-eight" suture or suture-mediated closure system.

Each delivery system has unique characteristics, which are described in detail elsewhere.[20,21] The Micra pacing capsule is preloaded in its delivery system, whereas the Aveir capsule has to be tethered to the docking cap on the delivery catheter via the docking button. The Micra is deployed by exerting forward catheter tip pressure such that the tines exit the device cup and engage the myocardium. The Aveir device is fixated with a screw-in mechanism necessitating 1 to 1.25 clockwise rotations of the device as evaluated by the radiopaque chevron maker on the device body without exerting tip pressure. The Micra device is released from the delivery catheter by cutting the tether and removing it. The Aveir tether cables are released from the anchoring points by rotating a small knob on the back end of the handle.

Recently, TLP implantations using surgical cutdown to the right or left internal jugular (IJ) vein or a percutaneous approach have been reported (**Fig. 6**).[10,22]

LEADLESS PACEMAKER CLINICAL DATA IN ADULT AND PEDIATRIC PATIENTS

Most clinical data describe use of TLP devices in adult patients (**Table 2**). The Micra system was associated with a 48% reduction in major complications when compared with the prespecified historical TV-PPM cohort.[2] The Micra Accelerometer Sensor Sub-Study (MASS) and MASS2 early feasibility studies showed that the Micra TIP can measure intracardiac accelerations caused by atrial contraction. The Micra Atrial Tracking Using a Ventricular Accelerometer (MARVEL) study demonstrated 87% AV synchrony during AV algorithm pacing in adults.[23]

The first report of TLP implantation in a pediatric patient with CHD was published by McCanta and colleagues[7] in 2018. Recently, a retrospective, nonrandomized, multicenter registry study designed to evaluate the safety and effectiveness of the Micra in children aged 21 years or less in a real-world setting was published.[12] During a mean follow-up period of 9.5 ± 5.3 months (30% of patients with follow-up > 12 months), there were 10 (16%) complications including one cardiac perforation/pericardial effusion, one nonocclusive femoral venous thrombus, and one retrieval and replacement of TLP due to high thresholds. There were no deaths, TLP infections, or device embolizations (see **Table 2**). Electrical parameters including capture thresholds, R wave sensing, and pacing impedances remained stable throughout follow-up.[12]

Despite encouraging results reported in the aforementioned pivotal trials, Hauser and colleagues[24] recently found an unexpected number of major adverse clinical events associated with TLP implantation in the FDA's Manufacturers and User Facility Device Experience database.

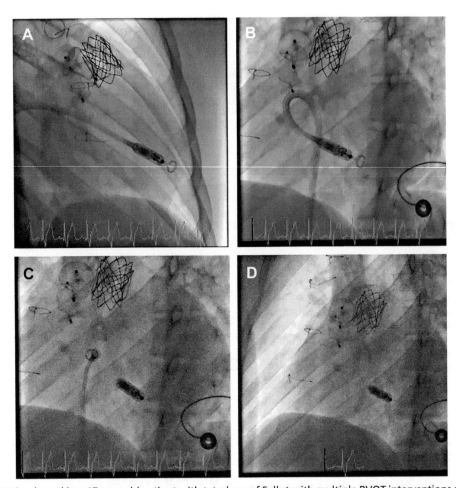

Fig. 5. TLP implanted in a 17-year old patient with tetralogy of Fallot with multiple RVOT interventions and intermittent high-grade AV block. The integrated Micra delivery system is used to access the right ventricle, as seen in this fluoroscopic video in an RAO and LAO views. Contrast is injected to confirm septal positioning of Micra device (A, B). To test fixation, a slow "pull-and-hold test" is performed with simultaneous cine angiography by slowly pulling on the tether system (C, D). The cine of RAO and LAO fluoroscopic views is reviewed frame by frame to assess tine engagement. If a tine is engaged in tissue, it will "splay" slightly open or begin to straighten out. Engagement of at least 2 tines and stable electrical measurements are mandatory to indicate adequate fixation before releasing the tether and removing the delivery system. AV, atrioventricular; LAO, left axial oblique; RAO, right axial oblique; RVOT, right ventricular outflow tract.

Although the overall incidence is low, TLP implantations may have a higher rate of myocardial and vascular perforations that result in cardiac tamponade and even death than had been previously reported.[24] Risk factors for perforation in adult patients are age greater than 85 years, body mass index less than 20 kg/m^2, female sex, heart failure, a non–atrial fibrillation indication, and chronic lung disease.[25] In pediatric patients, weight less than 30 kg was identified as a risk factor for major complications.[12]

LIMITATIONS OF LEADLESS PACING

The main limitations of TLP are the large-diameter implant sheaths, inability for long-term extraction of the Micra, lack of AV synchrony at faster heart rates, and limited long-term follow-up data. Battery longevity has been a concern in younger patients, although newer TLP versions offer improved battery longevity.[16]

LEADLESS PACING IN CONGENITAL HEART DISEASE
Benefits of Leadless Pacing in Congenital Heart Disease

Similar to the general population but magnified due to disease complexity and the need for frequent reinterventions, the most common CIED complications in patients with CHD are lead malfunction and generator pocket infections.[26–28]

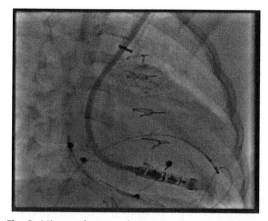

Fig. 6. Micra catheter and Micra implant via left internal jugular vein from AP view. AP, anteroposterior. (*From* Siddeek H, Alabsi S, Wong A, Cortez D. Leadless pacemaker implantation for pediatric patients through internal jugular vein approach: A case series of under 30 kg. Indian Pacing Electrophysiol J. 2023 Mar-Apr;23(2):39-44; with permission.)

Leadless pacing may therefore be a good solution in select patients. Clinical scenarios in which TLPs may be beneficial include:

1. Venous occlusion/obstruction

    Eliminating transvenous leads reduces the risk of chronic thrombosis and venous obstruction. TLPs can be implanted via either a femoral or IJ venous route as long as one of these is patent.[10,12,22]

2. Baffle obstruction

    Intracardiac baffle narrowing is not uncommon after certain types of CHD surgery. Obstruction in the superior limb of the systemic venous baffle of an atrial switch procedure, for example, is found in approximately 40% of cases, with a higher risk of hemodynamically significant obstruction associated with transvenous CIED leads.[29] Leadless pacing could decrease or eliminate the burden of intra-baffle leads.[30]

3. Subpulmonary AV valve abnormalities

    A lead crossing the AV valve may cause or worsen tricuspid regurgitation or stenosis[31]; it may preclude future transcatheter valve replacements without permanently jailing or extracting the pacing lead. Transvenous ventricular pacing is relatively contraindicated in patients with bioprosthetic TV (BTV), but the feasibility and safety of TLP through the BTV has been reported.[32]

4. Valvular endocarditis

    Endocardial leads have been reported to provide a substrate for pathogenic organisms and are associated with infectious endocarditis.[33] TLP technology may reduce the risk of valvular endocarditis.

5. Psychological benefits

    TLP imperceptibility to the patient offers mental and physical health benefits. Recovery after implant is simpler and shorter, with no shoulder/arm mobility limitations or additional surgical incisions to care for. Patients may engage in their usual activities relatively quickly after the procedure.

Table 2
Summary of adult and pediatric data for Food and Drug Administration-approved leadless pacemakers

	Micra IDE (n = 726) Adults Only	Micra PAR (n = 1871) Adults Only	Micra PACES Registry (n = 63) ≤21 y of Age Only	Aveir (n = 200) Adults Only
Implant success	99.2%	99.1%	98.4%	98%
Threshold @ implant (V@ ms)	0.63@0.24	0.63@0.24	0.77@0.24	0.85@0.4
Threshold @ follow up (F/U) (V@ ms)	0.54@0.24	0.66 @0.24	0.7@0.24	—
Complication rates	4%	2.7%	16%	4%
Pericardial effusion/ tamponade	1.5%	0.77%	1.6%	1.5%
Groin complications	0.7%	0.61%	6.25%	1%
Device dislodgement	0	0.5%	0	1%
Infection	0	0	0	0
Procedure-related deaths	0.13%	0.2%	0	0

6. TLP as a "bridge"

In some patients, delaying transvenous pacemaker implantation is of benefit for maintaining venous patency. TLP may be a reasonable temporary option because transvenous leads implanted in young patients are more difficult to manage long term and require complex lead extraction strategies.[34] The bridge strategy may be particularly beneficial in patients known to require a future cardiac surgical procedure during which the TLP can be surgically removed.

7. Existing transvenous pacing lead failure

In patients with transvenous pacing lead failure who are at high risk for lead extraction, it may be reasonable to cap and abandon the lead and perform a TLP implant.

8. Hybrid approaches

TLP hybrid approaches have been used. Needleman and colleagues[35] added a Micra AV in a 74-year-old patient with repaired tetralogy of fallot (TOF) who had a dual-chamber transvenous pacemaker with fractured RV pacing lead. The patient was able to have AV sequential pacing with AAI pacing via the transvenous device plus VDD pacing via the TLP after minimizing cross talk between the devices. A combination of ventricular pacing via TLP and defibrillation via S-ICD Boston Scientific Inc. (Marlborough, MA) has also been reported.[36]

Challenges of Leadless Pacing in Congenital Heart Disease

The ability to achieve successful implantation depends on a patient's anatomy and vascular access. Some patients may not have direct venous access to the heart. Patients with single ventricle physiology may not be eligible for TLP if there is no entry into the ventricle due to tricuspid atresia, patch closure of the AV valve, or a Fontan baffle. In patients with small RVs there may not be an adequate myocardial target for TLP implantation. There remains a risk for thrombus and systemic embolus and stroke in patients with single ventricle physiology or intracardiac shunts. Finally, current TLP systems are inadequate for patients with CHD with sinus node dysfunction who require atrial pacing and/or AV synchrony.

Real-World Data in Congenital Heart Disease

A summary of adult congenital heart disease (ACHD) cases reported in the literature is shown in **Table 3**.[30,37–46] Regarding children with CHD,

TLP implantation has only been reported in the subpulmonary ventricle in the absence of intracardiac shunts and in patients with biventricular physiology.[7,12,22] Implantation success and short-term electrical performance of TLP are similar to that reported in adult patients.[12] Complication rates seem to be similar, although there have been no reports of pericardial effusion/tamponade or deaths in the CHD population.[12]

Special Considerations for Leadless Pacing in Congenital Heart Disease

Multimodality imaging

Cardiac MRI or CT 3D reconstruction before TLP is useful in understanding segmental anatomy, subpulmonary ventricle size, AV valve anatomy, caval connections, and venous interruptions.[37] During the implantation procedure, the use of intracardiac or transesophageal echocardiography or 3D electroanatomic mapping with image integration may be useful.[42,47] RV angiography may also help to identify dense septomarginal trabeculations that may hinder a septal implant position and impede adequate TLP anchoring.[48]

Venous access

Preprocedural and/or intraprocedural imaging with angiography and/or duplex Doppler ultrasonography is useful in selecting venous site for TLP implantation. IJ veins are often larger than femoral veins and may accommodate the large introducer sheath more easily.[22] When using ultrasonography to assess the IJ veins, a Valsalva maneuver may be helpful to assess for stenosis.[10] For femoral vein cannulation, ultrasound-guided venous catheter cannulation is preferred to minimize groin complications.[21] Once femoral access is obtained, a venogram of the femoral and iliac vein should be performed to assess for stenosis or tortuosity that might interfere with advancement of the 27F introducer.

Interventional cardiology and cardiac surgery collaboration

Collaboration with interventional cardiology may be helpful especially if additional tools and techniques such as venoplasty, stenting, snaring, and baffle crossing are anticipated. Surgical cutdown for venous access may be preferred in some cases.[10]

Subpulmonary ventricle

The success of TLP implantation may depend on the morphology of the target ventricle. In a heavily trabeculated morphologic RV, it may be difficult to engage the myocardium. Conversely, in a morphologic LV, the smooth ventricular endocardium

Table 3
Summary of cases reported in literature of leadless pacing in ACHD

Authors/Year	N	CHD	Age (Years), Sex	Indication	Prior Pacemaker	Venous Access	TLP Device	Complications	Anticoagulation	Follow-up
Ferrero et al,[37] 2016	1	Single ventricle s/p class Glenn anastomosis	47 (F)	AV block	Yes	LFV	Micra VR	None	No	3 mo
Wilson et al,[38] 2016	1	Dextrocardia CCTGA	19 (F)	AV block	No	RFV	Micra VR	None	n/i	n/a
Sanhoury et al,[39] 2017	1	Dextrocardia DORV, VSD	47 (F)	AV block	Yes	LFV	Micra VR	None	n/i	n/a
Kotschet et al,[40] 2019	1	D-TGA s/p Mustard procedure	56 (M)	AV block	No	RFV	Micra VR	None	n/a	6 mo
Russell et al,[41] 2019	3	#1 ASD #2 VSD #3 ASD + VSD repair	88 (F) 22 (F) 63 (M)	SND SND AV block	No No No	RFV RFV LFV	Micra VR	None	No Yes n/i	7 mo 4 mo 1 mo
Dunne et al,[42] 2020	1	Single ventricle physiology Ebstein anomaly of TV	46 (F)	AV block	No	RFV	Micra VR	None	Yes	n/a
Rutland et al,[43] 2021	1	CCTGA	27 (F)	AV block	Yes	RFV	Micra AV	None	n/i	3 mo
Kautzner et al,[30] 2022	1	D-TGA s/p Mustard	48 (M)	AVB	Yes	RFV	Micra VR	None	n/i	4 mo
Ezhumalai and Singh Makkar,[44] 2022	1	AV canal defect, Eisenmenger syndrome, interrupted IVC	31 (F)	AV block	No	LFV	Micra VR	None	Yes	3
Mitchell et al,[45] 2022	2	D-TGA s/p Mustard	47(M) 49(M)	SND	No	LFV	Micra VR: implanted in left atrial appendage	None	n/i	n/a
Bassareo and Walsh,[46] 2022	15	Biventricular CHD = 12 Systemic RV = 2 Single ventricle = 1	37.5 ± 10.7 (M 53%)	SND: 9 AVB: 6	26.6%	n/a	Micra VR: 73% Micra AV: 27%	None	n/i	2.0 ± 0.3 y

Abbreviations: ASD, atrial septal defect; AV, atrioventricular; AVB, atrioventricular block; CCTGA, congenitally corrected transposition of the great arteries; D-TGA, dextro-transposition of the great arteries; DORV, double outlet right ventricle; F, Female; LFV, left femoral vein; M, male; n/a, not available; n/i, not indicated; RFV, right femoral vein; RV, right ventricle; SND, sinus node dysfunction; TV, tricuspid valve; VSD, ventricular septal defect.

may hinder passive fixation causing device dislodgement[49]; in active fixation, helical tipped TLP may be helpful in these cases.

Prior sternotomy

Cardiac perforation is the most catastrophic complication associated with TLP, and emergent surgical intervention can be lifesaving.[24] Although the potential for a life-threatening event in the setting of this complication should not be underestimated, fibrotic scar tissue in patients with prior sternotomies may obliterate the pericardial space and reduce blood loss. In this situation, however, cardiac perforations may directly exsanguinate into the thoracic cavity.[50] With an IJ venous approach, an superior vena cava (SVC) tear above the cardiac reflection may result in circulatory collapse. As is done in lead extraction procedures, it may be reasonable to perform TLP implantation with surgical backup.

Anticoagulation

There are sparse data regarding the frequency of postprocedure femoral or IJ venous occlusion. Venous thrombosis following use of a sheath this large may lead to thrombus and may preclude future venous access for cardiac procedures.[51] Clinical equipoise exists as to whether or not femoral venous thrombosis after cardiac catheterization in CHD warrants treatment,[52] and the decision to anticoagulate should be made on a case-by-case basis. In patients with single ventricle physiology or intracardiac shunts, anticoagulation should be strongly considered given the more significant consequences of venous thrombosis in these patients.[52]

Off-label use

It is important to acknowledge that TLP implantation in patients younger than 18 years, by nonfemoral routes and in nonstandard locations, is currently considered off-label. Reported nonstandard locations have included the subpulmonary LV, left atrial appendage, and epicardial right atrial appendage.[37,38,45,46,53] Informed consent and shared decision making should be discussed with patient and family.

SUMMARY

TLP offers potential benefits in children and adults with CHD, notably eliminating the complication risks of lead malfunction, venous occlusions, and pacemaker pocket infections. Although there may be technical challenges to implantation, with thoughtful patient selection, advanced planning, collaboration, and operator expertise, TLP can be successfully performed.

CLINICS CARE POINTS

- TLP offers benefits for patients with CHD, although not all patients are candidates. Patient selection, planning, and shared decision making are critical.

- Candidacy can be determined by understanding the type and frequency of pacing needed, venous anatomy, baffle patency, AV valve function, prior interventions performed, residual CHD lesions and shunts, anticipation for future cardiac surgery, and life expectancy.

- Advanced imaging may be helpful to verify candidacy and for procedural planning. Preprocedural 3-dimensional imaging, femoral or jugular venogram, and intraprocedural imaging tools including ventriculogram, transesophageal echocardiogram (TEE), intracardiac echocardiogram (ICE), and/or 3D electroanatomic image integration should be considered.

- Implant location should be anticipated, although operators should be prepared to modify this based on patient anatomy, pacing needs, and intracardiac obstacles.

- Collaboration with a surgeon and/or interventional cardiologist should be considered.

- Using an active fixation, helical-tipped TLP may help with implantation in smooth-walled left ventricles.

- TLP can be accomplished safely, efficiently, and effectively in patients with CHD, often under off-label indications and approaches, with elimination of the lead and generator pocket complications being common with epicardial and transvenous pacing systems.

DISCLOSURE

E.D. Sherwin: Clario (Bioclinica) consulting. M.J. Shah: Medtronic, Inc, Consultant.

SUPPLEMENTARY DATA

Supplementary data related to this article can be found online at https://doi.org/10.1016/j.ccep.2023.06.002.

REFERENCES

1. Duray GZ, Ritter P, El-Chami M, et al, Micra Transcatheter Pacing Study Group. Long-term performance of a transcatheter pacing system:12-Month results from the micra transcatheter pacing study. Heart Rhythm 2017;14:702–9.

2. Reynolds D, Duray GZ, Omar R, et al, Micra Transcatheter Pacing Study Group. A leadless intracardiac transcatheter pacing system. N Engl J Med 2016;374:533–41.

3. Ritter P, Duray GZ, Zhang S, et al, Micra Transcatheter Pacing Study Group. The rationale and design of the micra transcatheter pacing study: safety and efficacy of a novel miniaturized pacemaker. Europace 2015;17:807–13.

4. Roberts PR, Clementy N, Al Samadi F, et al. A leadless pacemaker in the real-world setting: the micra transcatheter pacing. system post-approval registry. Heart Rhythm 2017;14:1375–9.

5. El-Chami MF, Soejima K, Piccini JP, et al. Incidence and outcomes of systemic infections in patients with leadless pacemakers: data from the Micra IDE study. Pacing Clin Electrophysiol 2019;42(8): 1105–10.

6. El-Chami MF, Garweg C, Iacopino S, et al. Leadless pacemaker implant, anticoagulation status, and outcomes: results from the micra transcatheter pacing system post-approval registry. Heart Rhythm 2022; 19:228–34.

7. McCanta AC, Morchi GS, Tuozo F, et al. Implantation of a leadless pacemaker in a pediatric patient with congenital heart disease. HeartRhythm Case Rep 2018;4:506–9.

8. Breatnach CR, Dunne L, Al-Alawi K, et al. Leadless micra pacemaker use in the pediatric population: device implantation and short-term outcomes. Pediatr Cardiol 2020;41:683–6.

9. Gallotti RG, Biniwale R, Shannon K, et al. Leadless pacemaker placement in an 18-kilogram child: procedural approach and technical considerations. HeartRhythm Case Rep 2019;5:555–8.

10. Hackett G, Aziz F, Samii S, et al. Delivery of a leadless transcatheter pacing system as first-line therapy in a 28-kg pediatric patient through proximal right internal jugular surgical cutdown. J Innov Card Rhythm Manag 2021;12:4482–6.

11. Surti AK, Ambrose M, Cortez D. First description of a successful leadless pacemaker implantation via the left internal jugular vein (in a 20 kg patient). J Electrocardiol 2020;60:1–2.

12. Shah MJ, Borquez AA, Cortez D, et al. Transcatheter leadless pacing in children: a PACES collaborative study in the real-world setting. Circ Arrhythm Electrophysiol 2023;16(4):e011447.

13. Spickler JW, Rasor NS, Kezdi P, et al. Totally self-contained intracardiac pacemaker. J Electrocardiol 1970;3(3–4):325–31.

14. Reddy VY, Exner DV, Cantillon DJ, et al. Percutaneous implantation of an entirely intracardiac leadless pacemaker. N Engl J Med 2015;373(12): 1125–35.

15. Reddy VY, Exner DV, Doshi R, et al. LEADLESS II Investigators. Primary results on safety and efficacy

from the LEADLESS II-phase 2 Worldwide clinical trial. JACC Clin Electrophysiol 2022;8(1):115–7.

16. Escalante K. Micra AV2 and Micra VR2 longevity comparison. 2023. Medtronic Data on File.

17. Steinwender C, Khelae SK, Garweg C, et al. Atrioventricular synchronous pacing using a leadless ventricular pacemaker: results from the MARVEL 2 Study. JACC Clin Electrophysiol 2020;6:94–106.

18. Neugebauer F, Noti F, van Gool S, et al. Leadless atrioventricular synchronous pacing in an outpatient setting: early lessons learned on factors affecting atrioventricular synchrony. Heart Rhythm 2022; 19(5):748–56.

19. Heldon T, Escalante K, Fagan D. Device Longevity and AV Synchrony Algorithm Modeling of a Leadless Pacemaker Family: A Virtual Patient Analysis. January 2023. Medtronic Data on File.

20. Laczay B, Aguilera J, Cantillon DJ. Leadless cardiac ventricular pacing using helix fixation: Step-by-step guide to implantation. J Cardiovasc Electrophysiol 2023;34(3):748–59.

21. El-Chami MF, Roberts PR, Kypta A, et al. How to implant a leadless pacemaker with a tine-based fixation. J Cardiovasc Electrophysiol 2016;27(12):1495–501.

22. Siddeek H, Alabsi S, Wong A, et al. Leadless pacemaker implantation for pediatric patients through internal jugular vein approach: a case series of under 30 kg. Indian Pacing Electrophysiol J 2023;23(2): 39–44.

23. Chinitz L, Ritter P, Khelae SK, et al. Accelerometer-based atrioventricular synchronous pacing with a ventricular leadless pacemaker: results from the Micra atrioventricular feasibility studies. Heart Rhythm 2018;15(9):1363–71.

24. Hauser RG, Gornick CC, Abdelhadi RH, et al. Major adverse clinical events associated with implantation of a leadless intracardiac pacemaker. Heart Rhythm 2021;18(7):1132–9.

25. El-Chami MF, Al-Samadi F, Clementy N, et al. Updated performance of the Micra transcatheter pacemaker in the real-world setting: a comparison to the investigational study and a transvenous historical control. Heart Rhythm 2018; 15(12):1800–7.

26. Fortescue EB, Berul CI, Cecchin F, et al. Patient, procedural, and hardware factors associated with pacemaker lead failures in pediatrics and congenital heart disease. Hear Rhythm 2004;1:150–9.

27. Opić P, van Kranenburg M, Yap SC, et al. Complications of pacemaker therapy in adults with congenital heart disease: a multicenter study. Int J Cardiol 2013;168(4):3212–6.

28. Cohen MI, Bush DM, Gaynor JW, et al. Pediatric pacemaker infections: twenty years of experience. J Thorac Cardiovasc Surg 2002;124(4):821–7.

29. Bottega NA, Silversides CK, Oechslin EN, et al. Stenosis of the superior limb of the systemic venous

baffle following a Mustard procedure: an under-recognized problem. Int J Cardiol 2012;154:32–7.

30. Kautzner J, Wunschova H, Haskova J. Leadless pacemaker implant guided by intracardiac echocardiography in a patient after Mustard repair. Pacing Clin Electrophysiol 2022;45(4):571–3.

31. Addetia K, Harb SC, Hahn RT, et al. Cardiac implantable electronic device lead-Induced tricuspid regurgitation. JACC Cardiovasc Imaging 2019;12(4): 622–36.

32. Morani G, Bolzan B, Pepe A, et al. Leadless pacemaker through tricuspid bioprosthetic valve: early experience. J Arrhythm 2021;37(2):414–7.

33. Kołodzińska A, Kutarski A, Grabowski M, et al. Abrasions of the outer silicone insulation of endocardial leads in their intracardiac part: a new mechanism of lead-dependent endocarditis. EP Europace 2022;14(6):903–91.

34. Pham TDN, Cecchin F, O'Leary E, et al. Lead extraction at a pediatric/congenital heart disease center: the importance of patient age at implant. JACC Clin Electrophysiol 2022;8(3):343–53.

35. Needleman M, Symons J, Weber LA, et al. Novel use of an atrial sensing leadless pacemaker to treat complete heart block in a patient with repaired tetralogy of Fallot with pre-existing dual-chamber pacemaker with ventricular lead fracture. HeartRhythm Case Rep 2020;6:777–81.

36. Montgomery JA, Orton JM, Ellis CR. Feasibility of defibrillation and pacing without transvenous leads in a combined MICRA and S-ICD system following lead extraction. J Cardiovasc Electrophysiol 2017; 28(2):233–4.

37. Ferrero P, Yeong M, D'Elia E, et al. Leadless pacemaker implantation in a patient with complex congenital heart disease and limited vascular access. Indian Pacing Electrophysiol J 2016;16:201–4.

38. Wilson DG, Morgan JM, Roberts PR. Leadless pacing of the left ventricle in adult congenital heart disease. Int J Cardiol 2016;209:96–7.

39. Sanhoury M, Fassini G, Tundo F, et al. Rescue leadless pacemaker implantation in a pacemaker-dependent patient with congenital heart disease and no alternative routes for pacing. J Atr Fibrillation 2017;9(5):1542.

40. Kotschet E, Alasti M, Alison J. Micra implantation in a patient with transposition of great arteries. Pacing Clin Electrophysiol 2019;42(2):117–9.

41. Russell MR, Galloti R, Moore JP. Initial experience with transcatheter pacemaker implantation for adults with congenital heart disease. J Cardiovasc Electrophysiol 2019;30:1362–6.

42. Dunne L, Breatnach C, Walsh KP. Systemic ventricular implantation of a leadless pacemaker in a patient with a univentricular heart and atrioventricular node calcification. HeartRhythm Case Rep 2020;6: 265–7.

43. Rutland J, Tecson KM, Assar MD. Leadless ventricular pacemaker implant with atrial sensing in levo-transposition of the great arteries. HeartRhythm Case Rep 2021;7:220–3.

44. Ezhumalai B, Singh Makkar J. Transcatheter leadless permanent pacemaker in complex congenital heart disease with interrupted inferior vena cava: a challenging implantation. Indian Pacing Electrophysiol J 2022;22:165–8.

45. Mitchell AJ, Murphy N, Walsh KP. Fist in man implantation of a leadless pacemaker in the left atrial appendage following Mustard repair. Europace 2022;24:795.

46. Bassareo PP, Walsh KP. Micra pacemaker in adult congenital heart disease patients: a case series. J Cardiovasc Electrophysiol 2022;33:2335–43.

47. Martinez-Sande JL, Gonzalez-Melchor L, Garcia-Seara J, et al. Leadless pacemaker implantation with hybrid image mapping technique in a congenital heart disease case. HeartRhythm Case Rep 2021;7:797–800.

48. Garweg C, Vandenberk B, Foulon S, et al. Determinants of the difficulty of leadless pacemaker implantation. Pacing Clin Electrophysiol 2020;43:551–7.

49. Sterliński M, Demkow M, Plaskota K, et al. Percutaneous extraction of a leadless Micra pacemaker from the pulmonary artery in a patient with complex congenital heart disease and complete heart block. EuroIntervention 2018;14(2):236–7.

50. Tsang DC, Perez AA, Boyle TA, et al. Effect of prior sternotomy on outcomes in transvenous lead extraction. Circ Arrhythm Electrophysiol 2019;12(9): e007278.

51. Mahendran AK, Bussey S, Chang PM. Leadless pacemaker implantation in a four-year-old, 16-kg child. J Innov Card Rhythm Manag 2020;11(10): 4257–61.

52. Giglia TM, Massicotte MP, Tweddell JS, et al. Prevention and treatment of thrombosis in pediatric and congenital heart disease: a Scientific statement from the American heart association. Circulation 2013;128:2622–703.

53. Eltsov I, Sorgente A, de Asmundis C, et al. First in human surgical implantation of a leadless pacemaker on the epicardial portion of the right atrial appendage in a patient with a cardiac electronic devices mediated dermatitis. Interact Cardiovasc Thorac Surg 2022;35(1):ivac050.

Indications for Cardiac Resynchronization Therapy in Patients with Congenital Heart Disease

Peter P. Karpawich, MSc, MD, FHRS[a],*, Henry Chubb, MA, MBBS, PhD, FHRS[b,c]

KEYWORDS

- Congenital heart disease • Heart failure • Cardiac resynchronization • Biventricular pacing
- Conduction system/septal pacing

KEY POINTS

- Causes of heart failure in patients with congenital heart disease (CHD) typically differ from those in the elderly.
- Cardiac resynchronization therapy (CRT) pacing is applicable to patients with CHD but with many challenges.
- Evaluating CRT efficacy is still ongoing with no single definition of "responder."

INTRODUCTION

Although typically from different causes when compared with the elderly, children and patients with congenital heart defects (CHDs) can develop adverse or maladaptive geometric changes at the cardiac myocellular level. Regional areas of dyskinesia from structural anatomic variations, infarction, surgical procedures, infections, and chronic right ventricular (RV) apical pacing can alter contractility, leading to overall ventricular dysfunction. The resultant inter- and intraventricular dyssynchrony with myocellular alterations is frequently termed "remodeling" and contributes to clinical heart failure even at relatively early ages.[1,2]

Although perhaps not a panacea to completely normalize a dyssynchronous ventricle, cardiac resynchronization pacing therapy (CRT) using a biventricular lead implant approach and its related corollary of conduction system pacing (CSP) using a single lead implant are therapeutic interventions for treatment of and prevention of paced myocardial dysfunction. Together, CRT and CSP may be termed cardiac physiologic pacing (CPP); they can improve clinical well-being in general and can be an effective bridge to delay transplant among young patients with CHD with clinical heart failure.[3] As a pacing modality, CPP can be applied to young patients with both normal as well as diverse CHD anatomies (systemic RV, single ventricles). However, patients with CHD constitute a heterogeneous population with wide anatomic cardiac variations. As such, simple extrapolation of information from studies on older adults with normal cardiac anatomy is potentially counterproductive. Patients with CHD, at times, require more innovative approaches using epicardial or a combination of both epi- and endocardial stimulation, making CRT most challenging to achieve optimal efficacy (**Figs. 1–3**). The basic concept of CRT is that simultaneous stimulation of 2 separate ventricular regions can "reverse remodel" the altered

[a] Department of Pediatrics, Central Michigan University College of Medicine, Cardiac Electrophysiology, The Children's Hospital of Michigan, Detroit, MI, USA; [b] Stanford University School of Medicine, Stanford Medicine Children's Health, Palo Alto, CA, USA; [c] Pediatric Heart Center, 725 Welch Road, Suite 120, MC 5912, Palo Alto, CA 94304, USA
* Corresponding author. Pediatric Cardiology, 4th Floor Carls, The Children's Hospital of Michigan, 3901 Beaubien Boulevard, Detroit, MI 48201.
E-mail address: pkarpawi@dmc.org

Card Electrophysiol Clin 15 (2023) 433–445
https://doi.org/10.1016/j.ccep.2023.07.005

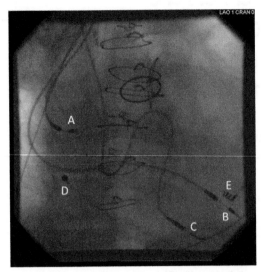

Fig. 1. Fluoroscopic view of CRT lead positions in a patient with CHD with repaired L-TGA/VSD and RV to pulmonary artery conduit. A: atrial; B: right ventricle; C: coronary sinus; D: abandoned atrial; E: ventricular epicardial pacing leads.

ventricular muscle alignments and improve function by changing contractility stress forces.[4] CSP may be a more physiologic approach but is in its infancy in terms of evidence in CHD and almost universally requires an endovascular approach.

This article focuses largely on CRT; CSP is discussed in detail in Jeremy P. Moore and Aarti S.

Dalal's article, "Conduction System Pacing for Patients with Congenital Heart Disease," in this issue. However, specific recommendations for CPP (encompassing both CRT and CSP) have recently been published by the Heart Rhythm Society.[5] Some of these indications do not explicitly differentiate between CRT and CSP, and therefore this article refers to CPP when this is the case. This first section discusses issues associated with CRT as a therapeutic modality: clinical efficacy, contractility responses, and lead implant concerns. The second section discusses available guidelines, past and present clinical applications and evidence, and specific concerns as applied to patients with CHD.

Section 1: Cardiac Resynchronization Concepts

Cardiac resynchronization therapy evolution

At the onset of therapeutic cardiac pacing, initial concerns were both to reestablish a normal heart rate and to assure pacing lead integrity and stability. As a result, the right atrial appendage and ventricular apex became "traditional" lead implant sites with limited concern for contractility response. However, with increasing applications of cardiac pacing to children and patients with repaired CHD and the anticipation of the need for decades-long pacing, adverse effects on myocellular structure and contractility (pacing-induced cardiomyopathy [PICM]) became evident.[6,7] Improved lead designs and delivery systems resulted in a more hemodynamically guided lead

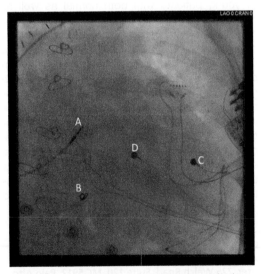

Fig. 2. Fluoroscopic view of CRT leads applied as a combination transvenous/epicardial system in a patient with CHD with a single ventricle/Fontan procedure. A: transvenous atrial; B: epicardial anterior ventricular position; C: epicardial posterior ventricular position; D: abandoned fractured epicardial atrial.

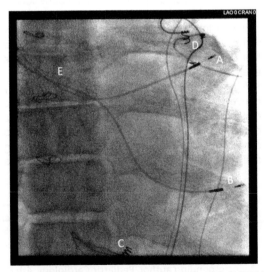

Fig. 3. CRT leads in a patient with CHD with D-TGA/Mustard. A: left atrial; B: left ventricle; C: epicardial right ventricle; D: abandoned epicardial leads; E: atrial baffle stent.

implant approach introduced as "Alternate/Select Site" pacing (ie, nonapical lead implant).[8] Later clinical applications demonstrating hemodynamic advantages evolved to the current concept of CSP based on septal lead implant that approximates regions of the proximal ventricular conduction system; this now includes "optimized septal" pacing, direct/indirect "His bundle pacing" (HBP), and "left bundle branch area pacing" (LBBAP). Pacing from these selective septal implant sites is typically associated with more normalized contractility responses and QRS configurations in deference to apical sites. As a result, the terms "CSP/CPP" now comprise the latest iteration of the older historical term, "physiologic pacing" previously associated with rate-response as well as atrioventricular (AV) synchrony.[9,10] Because lead implant with concomitant contractility measurements can assure optimized mechanical response, selective septal sites may theoretically prevent pacing-induced myopathy or improve existing dyssynchrony as a form of single-site ventricular CRT.[11] However, there are limited definitive clinical studies that compare sites among patients with CHD. Simultaneous stimulation from 2 separate ventricular sites was initially coined "biventricular" pacing (BiV, BVP) and initiated a new era of improving clinical heart failure by altering contractile forces of a failing/dyssynchronous ventricle even among patients with CHD.[12,13] Because a failing ventricle was considered "desynchronized," dual-site pacing was termed "cardiac resynchronization therapy" (CRT), although actual "resynchronization" is often a somewhat ambiguous and ill-defined concept.

Ventricular contractility, normal versus paced

Based on the geometry of a prolate spheroid (think American football shape), left ventricular (LV) contractility involves shortening as well as twisting and torsion of endo- and epicardial myofibers in opposite (clockwise-counterclockwise) directions. Contraction involves predominately a reduction in the transverse chamber diameter. In contradistinction, the RV contracts more in a base-to-apex pattern with minimal free wall to septum movement. This difference contributes to the development of early heart failure among some patients with CHD with systemic RVs.[11] With normal AV node conduction, the proximal LV septum activates initially, followed by the RV 5 to 10 msec later, supporting the concept of lead implant in this proximal septal area if ventricular conduction is intact. Altered muscle strain and sheer forces due to regional dyskinesis or pacing can change normal endo- to epicardial electrical activation and mechanical cellular responses. Studies of ventricular contractility using directly measured pressure-volume loops and contractility indices (dP/dt) at various stimulation sites have demonstrated the importance of selective lead implant in myocardial response.[14–16] In patients with an intrinsic left bundle branch block (LBBB), stimulation distal to the site of block (left bundle pacing) can potentially activate the normal distal conduction system, resulting in improved QRS and contractility as the most recent form of single-site CRT.[17] However, an intrinsic LBBB QRS pattern seldom occurs among young patients or patients with CHD. It is important to recognize that not all LBBB patterns are equal. An intrinsic LBBB QRS pattern exhibits different LV electrical activation and contraction patterns from an LBBB QRS morphology caused by RV apical pacing.[18] Therefore, simple extrapolation of study results from patients with ischemic LBBB to those with pacing-induced LBBB can be counterproductive. As indicated earlier, although selective septal pacing is beneficial, definitive data on benefits of specific His bundle or left bundle pacing in patients with CHD are lacking. The recommendation for CRT lead implant at the area of latest LV activation also may not apply to patients with CHD with a pacing-created LBBB QRS.[19] Because there is no universal "best implant site" applicable to all patients, especially among those with repaired CHD, lead implant based on some specific contractility responses (eg, pressure-time [dP/dt], strain, pressure-volume loops), in addition to standard lead threshold/sensing issues, may be beneficial. Comparable with the need for optimal shock vectors for ICDs, dual CRT lead placements will dictate resultant stimulation and contraction sequences (**Fig. 4**). As a result, although a patient may have biventricular stimulation, actual contractility responses can vary without any positive clinical or hemodynamic results.

Biventricular versus resynchronization pacing/cardiac resynchronization therapy efficacy

As a basic premise, not all CRT is BiV and not all BiV pacing is CRT. If CRT stimulation consistently improved contractility/synchronization, then all patients should be "responders." However, the reported 30% to 50% "nonresponder" rates raise an obvious question of "why?" Proposed reasons include degree of heart failure, underlying anatomic issues, improper device programming, and clinical comorbidities. However, ineffective lead implant site of stimulation is a prime reason.[20] To compensate for this latter factor, multiple point pacing to improve contractility vectors has been proposed.[21] Another concern in reporting CRT efficacy has been the diverse definitions of success,

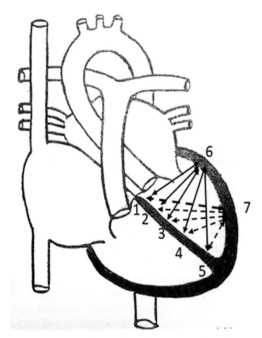

Fig. 4. Schematic representation of LV CRT stimulation and resultant contractility vectors from potential paired RV[1–5] and coronary sinus[6,7] lead implant sites. Contractility vectors change in relation to stimulation sites, and ineffective lead positioning contributes to nonresponder rates.

which have included reduced mortality from any cause, any improvement in clinical New York Heart Association (NYHA) classification, improved quality-of-life surveys (irrespective of any placebo effect), a simple 5% ejection fraction (EF) change, or any QRS duration shortening. Most reported studies do not directly measure contractility response but rely on indirect parameters of electrical activation (QRS duration) or chamber volumes (EF) and equate those to mechanical contractility, which is questionable.[22,23] Unfortunately, EF measurement techniques (eg, shortening fraction derivation, Simpson method) are often not specified among CRT publications, leading to interpretation difficulty. Although these measures provide some estimation of overall global ventricular volumes, regional wall motion abnormalities, which are particularly common in patients with repaired CHD, often negate EF accuracy. However, more updated echocardiographic parameters have shown improved correlations with contractility. In a recent study by Menon and colleagues change in global longitudinal strain was the only echo parameter among 10 measured values that corresponded with clinical and direct hemodynamically measured contractility improvements in younger patients with and without repaired CHD.[24] QRS

duration shortening has also not had a consistent correlation with CRT efficacy, at times increasing despite clinical improvements[25,26]; this reflects the differences between electrical and mechanical synchrony. The only patient subgroup in which QRS duration shortening seems to correlate with a positive CRT response has been patients with CHD with preexisting pacemakers.[24]

Section 2: Clinical Applications

Current guidelines

The indications for CRT (and CSP) are entwined with the complexity of the individual case in a manner that is more complex than most CRT cases in the structurally normal heart. Techniques for implant are discussed in detail in the next article, but, clearly, the indication for CRT in every patient is an individualized risk/benefit assessment. Dogmatic guidelines are therefore challenging to define, and indeed are probably inappropriate in many cases, but there are numerous sets of guidelines that refer to CRT in CHD in varying degrees of detail. In addition, the recently published 2023 Heart Rhythm Society Guidelines for physiologic pacing (in both structurally normal heart and CHD) provide new and more definitive guidance.[5]

An important further consideration is the need for optimal medical management of heart failure symptoms before CRT. There are no explicit recommendations in the CHD or non-CHD guidelines for the length of time that this should be maintained before implant. However, it is clear that a trial of pharmacologic therapy is appropriate before pursuing an invasive and complex therapy such as CRT. In the context of the limited evidence available for patients with CHD, at least 1 month of pharmacologic treatment would be consistent with the inclusion criteria of major non-CHD trials such as COMPANION.[27]

2023 Cardiac Physiologic Pacing guidelines Before the publication of the 2023 CPP guidelines, most sets of guidelines had distinguished between pediatric and adult patients with CHD.[5] The new guidelines are outlined in **Table 1** and **Fig. 5A** and take a more anatomic-based, rather than age-based, approach. There is no longer a Class 1 indication for CPP in CHD, but the main Class 2a recommendation for CPP has broader parameters for consideration of CPP in those with systemic LV. In contrast to the Class 1 indication of the 2014 PACES/HRS Consensus Statement on Management of Arrhythmias in CHD[28] (systemic LV, LVEF $\leq$ 35%, LBBB, QRS $\geq$ 150 ms, and NYHA class II–IV), the degree of dysfunction for consideration is now LVEF less than 45%. In addition,

Table 1
Recommendations for cardiac physiologic pacing in patients with congenital heart disease

Class of Recommendation	Level of Evidence	Recommendation
2a	C - LD	In patients with CHD on GDMT with a *systemic LV*, LVEF <45%, and ventricular dyssynchrony (as defined by a QRS duration z score of >+3 or ventricular pacing >40%), CRT with BVP is reasonable to reduce the risk of mortality or need for transplant.
2a	C - LD	In patients with CHD and a *systemic single ventricle* who require pacing, apical pacing is reasonable in preference to nonapical pacing.
2b	C - LD	In patients with CHD and a *systemic single ventricle with symptomatic HF* on GDMT, CRT with multisite ventricular pacing may be considered to maintain functional class or ventricular function.
2b	C - LD	In patients with CHD and a *systemic RV* with symptomatic HF on GDMT associated with ventricular electrical delay or requiring substantial ventricular pacing, CRT with BiV pacing may be considered to improve or maintain functional class or ventricular function.
2b	C - LD	In patients with CHD and a *subpulmonary RV* with RV dysfunction and RBBB, CRT with fusion-based pacing may be considered to improve RV function.
2b	C - LD	In patients with *ccTGA and AV block* in whom anatomic repair has not been performed, CSP with HBP or LBBAP may be considered to improve functional status.

Abbreviations: BiV, biventricular; ccTGA, congenitally corrected transposition of the great arteries; CSP, conduction system pacing; GDMT, guideline-directed medical therapy; HBP, His bundle pacing; HF, heart failure; LBBAP, left bundle branch area pacing; LD, limited data.
Adapted from the 2023 HRS/APHRS/LAHRS guideline on cardiac physiologic pacing for the avoidance and mitigation of heart failure.[5]

rather than a strict requirement for broad LBBB (which is relatively rarely encountered in CHD), a more global marker of electrical dyssynchrony (QRS duration z-score >+3 or ventricular pacing >40%) has replaced it. It should also be noted that most of the current recommendations across the differing CHD anatomies are explicitly for CRT rather than CSP.

Patients with congenital heart disease with bradycardia pacing indication or pacing-induced cardiomyopathy For many, if not the majority, of CHD CRT recipients, there is already an underlying bradycardia pacing indication, and CRT is performed in the context of a high ventricular pacing burden. Implant for correction of electrical dyssynchrony alone (such as bundle branch block) is relatively rare.[29,30] Upgrade to CRT for management of PICM is widely accepted as a strong indication for CRT, with high response rates observed.[28,31,32]

However, the decision for implant of a CRT system at initial implant is more challenging. The 2023 CPP guidelines do not directly address the question except for pediatric patients in general, in

whom a Class 2a recommendation is made for targeting lower risk pacing sites (RV midseptal, inflow or outflow tract for transvenous, and apical LV [systemic ventricle] for epicardial systems) (**Fig. 5**B).

The 2014 PACES/HRS Consensus Statement places a Class 2a recommendation for CRT in adults with CHD and high (>40%) anticipated ventricular pacing, but only for those with reduced ventricular function (systemic ventricular EF [SVEF] ≤35%).[28] It is likely that many more patients stand to benefit from more physiologic pacing, particularly in patient cohorts such as those with a single ventricle in whom pacing-associated morbidity and mortality seems particularly high.[33] More routine use of CSP, if a transvenous approach is possible for the individual patient, is likely to emerge, but the evidence is currently limited.

Comparison of new cardiac physiologic pacing guidelines with other congenital heart disease and heart failure guidelines The section of the 2023 CPP guidelines on CHD indications is relatively succinct. As with most medical guidelines,

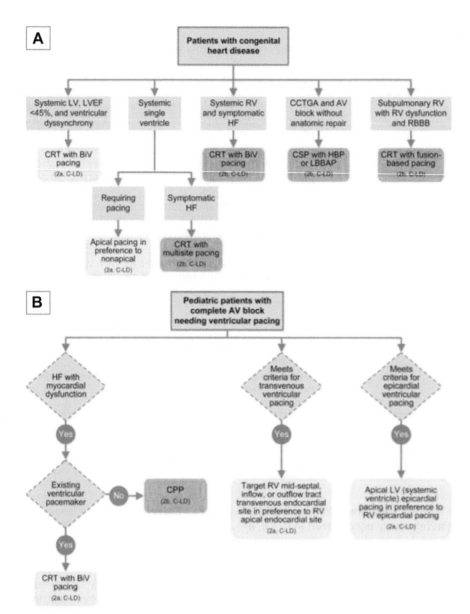

Fig. 5. Overview of recommendations for cardiac physiologic pacing in patients with CHD (*A*) and pediatric (*B*) patients. Note that the pediatric guidelines refer explicitly to patients without CHD. (Adapted with permission from the 2023 HRS/APHRS/LAHRS guideline on cardiac physiologic pacing for the avoidance and mitigation of heart failure.[5])

there are occasions when older, but more detailed, guidelines may proscribe a management strategy for a specific clinical scenario that is not addressed in the most recent guidelines. However, there are minimal conflicts due to the abbreviated nature of prior guidelines.

The 2014 PACES/HRS Consensus Statement on Management of Arrhythmias in CHD were by far the most comprehensive.[28] They created a relatively complex decision tree for CRT in patients with adult congenital heart disease (ACHD), and

the main changes are outlined earlier. The rest of the guidelines leave a great deal of latitude for clinician discretion. The 2018 AHA/ACC Guidelines for the management of patients with ACHD do not discuss CRT,[34] and the 2022 AHA/ACC/HFSA Heart Failure Guidelines do not discuss CHD in their thorough review of CRT.[31] From a European perspective, the 2021 ESC ACHD guidelines simply suggest that indications for CRT (or HBP) in patients with a biventricular circulation and systemic LV should follow "standard" criteria. However, for other patient groups, guidance was deferred with the statement that further research is required.[35] The 2022 ESC Guidelines on Cardiac Pacing and CRT take a similar nonprescriptive approach, stating that standard indications may be considered but that in general in CHD "…multidisciplinary teams in experienced centers should be involved in the decision-making process."[36]

For pediatric patients with CHD there has been even less prior guidance regarding the indications for CRT. In 2014, the ISHLT Pediatric Heart and Lung Transplant guidelines reviewed pediatric indications for CRT.[37] Echoing the ACHD guidelines, a Class 2a indication was defined for patients with a systemic LV, an EF less than 35%, complete LBBB, and QRS duration (native or paced) longer than the upper limit of normal for age and NYHA class II to IV. Class 2b indications were defined for patients with similar criteria as those with a systemic RV (with right bundle branch block [RBBB] rather than LBBB) and those with a single ventricle with either an LBBB or RBBB QRS pattern. The 2021 PACES Expert Consensus Statement on CIEDSs deliberately excluded CRT/CPP, given the planned physiologic pacing guidelines.[38]

Evidence for cardiac resynchronization therapy in congenital heart disease

Multiple large prospective randomized controlled trials have demonstrated that CRT improves morbidity and mortality for non-CHD adults with heart failure.[39–44] However, patients with CHD were excluded from all prospective randomized trials. As a result, evidence for the use of CRT in the CHD population relies on retrospective cohort studies. **Table 2** outlines those studies that have assessed the outcomes for CRT (or CSP) in 20 or more patients with CHD. These studies span multiple eras in the evolution of CRT, with a great deal of patient and device heterogeneity.[29,30,32,45–51]

Markers for response to CRT, as discussed earlier, are generally challenging but never more so than among patients with CHD. Cohort studies have generally demonstrated relatively high response rates in this high morbidity cohort but with multiple different definitions of success used. More recently, propensity score–matched studies have sought to establish whether CRT response may be assessed against more robust outcomes such as transplant-free survival. The reliability of any analysis heavily depends on correct identification and phenotyping of controls, but it is highly promising that studies have demonstrated an association between CRT and survival. Such studies have used inclusion criteria of SVEF less than or equal to 45%, significant electrical dyssynchrony (defined as QRS duration z-score >+3 or

ventricular pacing >40%), and symptomatic heart failure.[29] However, further studies are clearly required to corroborate these results using alternative methods, ideally prospectively.

The merits of conduction system pacing versus multisite cardiac resynchronization therapy Conventional CRT with 2 pacing sites achieves CRT through nonphysiological fusion of paced wavefronts from at least 2 ventricular pacing locations. CSP may represent a more physiologic approach and can be advantageous both in patients with a bradycardia pacing indication as well as those with dyssynchrony. CSP is discussed in detail in Jeremy P. Moore and Aarti S. Dalal's article, "Conduction System Pacing for Patients with Congenital Heart Disease," in this issue, but pertinent to the indications for conventional, 2-site, CRT in CHD is the consideration of the alternative CPP modalities. Unfortunately, to date, there are no definitive studies comparing paced contractility responses or chronic clinical outcomes between CSP and conventional CRT in pediatric patients or patients with CHD, let alone the role of His-optimized CRT and LBBAP-optimized CRT.[52]

In the non-CHD adult patient, studies have sought to establish whether CSP may be superior to BVP. A 2022 multicenter observational study of CSP versus BVP was performed by Vijayaraman and colleagues, assessing a primary outcome of heart failure hospitalization or death in 477 (BVP: n = 219, CSP: n = 258) consecutive patients (mean age 72 ± 12 y). All patients had LVEF less than or equal to 35% and Class 1 or 2 indications for CRT, and there was a significantly lower incidence of the primary outcome in the CSP cohort (28% vs 38%; hazard ratio 1.52; P = .013). However, because of study design and patient comorbidities, the investigators conclude that results "should be interpreted with some degree of caution."[53]

In patients with CHD, Moore and colleagues also examined the potential superiority of CSP over BVP on assessment of a subset of their 65 CSP patients (mean age 37 ± 21 years; 46 [96%] with AV block) across 7 centers.[30] Propensity score matching to a BVP CRT cohort was performed for a subset of 25 patients with similar baseline characteristics. Change in LVEF was similar but the decrease in QRS duration was greater in the CSP cohort with similar complication rates.

Predictors of response to cardiac resynchronization therapy

In the balancing of risk/benefit, the identification of markers for likely response to CRT in patients with CHD would be extremely helpful. The strongest predictors of response to CRT in adult patients

Table 2
Publications including at least 20 patients with congenital heart disease receiving cardiac resynchronization therapy

	Dubin et al,[47] 2005	Janousek et al,[38] 2009	Cecchin et al,[48] 2009	Sakaguchi et al,[49] 2015	Karpawich et al,[3] 2017	Flügge et al,[50] 2018	Koyak et al,[51] 2018	Leyva et al,[52] 2019	Chubb et al,[36] 2020	Cano et al,[53] 2021	Moore et al,[37] 2022
Single/Multicenter	Multi	Multi	Single	Single	Single	Multi	Multi	Single	Single	Multi	Multi
Total patients, n	103	109	60	20	26	55	48	23	63[a]	20	65
Age, (Median/Average), y	13 (0.3–55)	17 (0.3–74)	15 (0.4–47)	22 (10–32)	23 (4–39)	21 (8.7–38)	47 (18–74)	42 ± 14	11 (3–25)	32 ± 17	37 ± 21
Follow-up duration (mo)	4 (0.6–12)	Median 7.5	8 (0.1–63)	Median 6	46 (4–144)	83 (38–121)	31 (1–106)	49 (26–73)	33 (10–73)	16 (7–19)	12
CHD population, n (%)	73 (71)	87 (80)	46 (77)	20 (100)	26 (100)	55 (100)	48 (100)	23 (100)	51 (81)	20 (100)	65 (100)
Type of CRT system, n (%)											
Epicardial	48 (47)	36 (33)	38 (63)	...	2 (7)	27 (50)	9 (19)	3 (13)	43 (68)	0	0
Transvenous	45 (44)	45 (41)	17 (28)	...	17 (65)	28 (50)	37 (77)	20 (87)	17 (27)	0	0
Hybrid	10 (10)	28 (26)	5 (8)	...	5 (19)	0	2 (42)	0	3 (5)	0	0
CRT-D	20 (20)	20 (18)	15 (25)	2 (10)	2 (97)	6 (11)	38 (79)	6 (26)	19 (30)	0	0
CSP (HBP/LBBP/LVSP)	0	0	0	0	—	0	0	0	0	10/5/5	17/38/10
Pre-CRT NYHA Class	39 (38%) III or IV	Median 2.5 III or IV	2 [1–3]	2 [2–2.25]	7 (II) 18 (III-IV)	...	35 (73%) III or IV	3 [2–3]	2 [2–3]	1 [1–2]	...
Pre-CRT QRS duration (ms)	166 ± 33	Median 160	149 (95–210)	183 ± 28	153 ± 32 65% prepaced	...	181 ± 33	171 ± 31	159 ± 35	144 ± 32	142 ± 37
LBBB	...	10 (9)	10 (17)	...	Prepaced only	...	12 (25)	15 (65)	43 (68)[b]	...	...
Pre-CRT sysV EF (%)	26 ± 12	Median 27	36 (8–70)	34 ± 11	30 ± 8	...	44 (92%) <35%	33 ± 13	32 ± 8	50 ± 14	50 ± 14
Outcomes After CRT											
Definition of Response	Any increase in SVEF	↓ NYHA class by ≥ 1 class or Any increase in SVEF	↑SVEF by 10% proportion	Not defined	↑ dP/dt >15% ↓ NYHA class by ≥ 1 Transplant free	Not defined	↓ NYHA class by ≥ 1 class or ↑SVEF by ≥ 1 class	Not defined	Improved survival vs matched controls	Change in SVEF	Change in SVEF
Systemic LV and Biventricular Circulation											
Total number (%)	79 (79)	69 (63)	38 (63)	7 (35)	16 (62)	42 (76)	37 (77)	12 (52)	44 (51)	13 (65)	65 (100)
Of whom CHD (% of systemic LVs)	49 (62)	47 (68)	26 (68)	7 (100)	16 (100)	42 (100)	37 (100)	12 (100)	32 (73)	13 (100)	65 (100)
Nonresponders	2 (3)	11/54 (20)	....	... (EF 36→40, P<.01)	0	...	6 (16)	...	HR 0.26 (0.11–0.61)	... (EF 54→58, P=.04)	... (ΔEF +9.0%)

Systemic RV and Biventricular Circulation

Number (%)	17 (17)	27	9	7 (35)	8 (31)	13 (24)	11 (23)	9 (39)	10 (20)	7 (35)	0
Nonresponders	4/17 (23)	3/22 (14)	6/9 (66)	… (EF 36→36.5, P = .45)	0	…	5 (45)	…	HR 0.14 (0.02–0.92)	… (EF 40→44, P = .01)	…
Inferior to LV resynchronization?	No	Borderline	Likely Yes	Yes	No	Unknown	No	Unknown	No	No	N/A
	Improvement observed in EF or clinical status	No difference vs sysLV except ΔSVEDD z-score	No formal comparison: high nonresponder rate, but very different patient substrate	No significant improvement in EF or EDVI	All pts preselected for CRT based on acute CRT pacing response	Minimal follow-up data. One death in each of sysLV and sysRV groups	Non-significant trend (P = .16) to increased proportion of sysRV in non-responders	No breakdown	Significantly reduced rate of transplant/death	Both showed significant improvement in EF	N/A

Single Ventricle

Number (%)	7 (7)	4 (4)	13	6 (30)	2 (7)	2 (4)	0	2 (9)	9 (18)	0	0
Nonresponders	5 (71)	1/4 (25)	1/13 (8)	… (EF 29→33, P<.01)	0	1 (50)	N/A	…	HR 0.26 (0.03–2.1)	N/A	N/A
Inferior to LV resynchronization?	Yes	No	Likely no	No	No	Unknown	N/A	Unknown	Likely no	N/A	N/A
	No change in EF	No association with nonresponse	No formal comparison, but low nonresponder rate	A significant improvement observed in EF and EDVI	All pts preselected for CRT based on acute CRT pacing response	Low patient numbers. One died at Fontan conversion	N/A	No breakdown	Nonsignificant trend to improved outcome	N/A	N/A

Numbers are presented as mean ± standard deviation, median (range) or median [25th–75th quartiles].

Abbreviations: CRT-D, CRT-defibrillator; CSP, conduction system pacing; EF, ejection fraction; HBP, his bundle pacing; HTx, heart transplant; LBBB, left bundle branch block; LBBP, left bundle branch pacing; LVSP, LV septal pacing; NYHA, New York Heart Association; QRSd, QRS duration; RBBB, right bundle branch block; sysLV, systemic left ventricular; sysRV, systemic right ventricular; sysV, systemic ventricular.

a CRT subjects propensity score matched to controls.
b Conduction delay to the lateral wall of the systemic ventricle.

with structurally normal hearts are an LBBB morphology and QRS duration greater than or equal to 150 msec. More advanced measures of electrical and mechanical dyssynchrony have generally struggled to outperform these simple indices.[54,55] However, in CHD, surface electrocardiogram morphology is frequently not a strong indicator of the exact underlying cause of electrical dyssynchrony, such as a bundle branch block. There are, although, early data that apparent conduction delay to the lateral wall of the systemic ventricle (such as an LBBB pattern in a repaired simple ventricular septal defect or an RBBB pattern in dextro-transposition of the great arteries [d-TGA] postatrial switch) may be associated with an improved CRT response, simplifying the quantification of dyssynchrony.[29,56,57]

There is also the factor of cardiac morphology that could play an important role in CRT response. However, **Table 2** outlines the results of CRT/CSP in patients with systemic right or single ventricles compared with those with biventricular systemic left ventricles, and there are conflicting results across studies. CRT responses have been observed in all groups, and there seems to be no single cardiac morphology that precludes CRT application. However, in considering the individualized indication for CRT, the impact of underlying CHD and risk/benefit should always be evaluated.[5]

Biventricular circulation with systemic right ventricle The patient group with biventricular circulation and a systemic RV morphology mainly comprise the aging population with d-TGA who have undergone an intra-atrial baffle procedure (Mustard/Senning) and those with congenitally corrected or levo-TGA. The response to CRT is particularly challenging to assess in the more complex morphology of the RV, and studies looking at hard outcomes such as transplant or death have generally identified a less positive response.[29] However, the clinical time course of deterioration in the systemic RV patient is often more rapid, and simply delaying deterioration may itself represent a strong response to CRT.

Single ventricle pacing Single ventricle patients seem to be at a markedly increased risk of PICM, and therefore, CRT holds particular attraction in an aim to mitigate that risk.[33] Studies of CRT in this population have demonstrated an improvement in SVEF and contractility but no consistent survival benefit.[29,58] The indication for CRT in single ventricle patients is complicated by the need to avoid transvenous ventricular leads, which currently almost completely mandates an epicardial approach, although a hybrid approach with a transvenous coronary sinus lead implant for posterior ventricular stimulation (CS-V) combined with an anterior epicardial V lead is technically feasible in select anatomies. Pacing among such patients is made more challenging in view of multiple prior sternotomies that occur in almost all cases. Data would therefore suggest that preemptive placement of a multisite (CRT) pacing system should be considered in single ventricle patients with a high anticipated pacing burden.

Resynchronization of the subpulmonary right ventricle Data regarding resynchronization of the subpulmonary ventricle with an RBBB QRS pattern, such as the failing RV in tetralogy of Fallot, are scarce. Studies have demonstrated positive acute and short-term (6 months) CRT pacing responses.[59,60] The more technically straightforward approach of single-site RV pacing at the location of latest ventricular activation may also be performed. Janousek and colleagues demonstrated significant improvement in functional indices with single-site RV pacing in 6 patients with CHD (3 with concomitant surgery), aiming for fusion of activation with the spontaneous wave front in order to mitigate the risk of discoordinate LV contraction.[59] However, the achievement of optimal fusion across a wide range of heart rates is challenging and has not been replicated by other investigators.[60,61]

SUMMARY

CRT is an important therapeutic tool in the management of cardiac failure. When targeted correctly, reversing clinically important electromechanical dyssynchrony, the impact on the clinical course for patients with CHD can be profound. However, the heterogeneity of the CHD patient group, challenges in defining optimal CRT modality and timing, and varying assessment of response frequently result in a clinical decision-making process clouded by highly individualized risks and benefits. This article has outlined some of the considerations when deliberating the implant of a CRT system, including the physiologic mechanisms, guidelines, and clinical evidence. CSP may change some of these factors profoundly, but with a patient-tailored approach, implementation of CRT in CHD is an increasingly vital tool in the management of the failing heart with CHD.

CLINICS CARE POINTS

- CPP is a term that encompasses both conventional, multisite CRT and newer CSP.

- Acute indices of response to CRT, such as change in dP/dt, may assist in lead placement or patient selection.
- Assessment of chronic response to CRT is highly challenging in the heterogenous CHD population, and there is no single parameter accepted as a marker of response.
- The recent 2023 Cardiac Physiologic Pacing Guidelines have provided new guidance on the indications for CRT, with a less severe EF threshold (45%) and more general electrical dyssynchrony threshold (QRS duration z-score >+3).
- CSP is likely to become an increasingly prevalent method of implementing resynchronization, with early studies suggesting outcomes at least as good as conventional CRT in some populations.
- Retrospective studies of CRT in CHD suggest that there is currently no cardiac morphology (such as systemic RV or single V) that is a consistent predictor of worse or better response to CRT.

DISCLOSURE

P.P. Karpawich, H. Chubb: None.

REFERENCES

1. Shaddy RE, George AT, Jaecklin T, et al. Systematic Literature review on the incidence and prevalence of heart failure in children and Adolescents. Pediatr Cardiol 2018;39(3):415–36.
2. McKay RG, Pfeffer MA, Pasternak RC, et al. Left ventricular remodeling after myocardial infarction: a corollary to infarct expansion. Circulation 1986; 74(4):693–702.
3. Karpawich PP, Bansal N, Samuel S, et al. 16 Years of cardiac resynchronization pacing among congenital heart disease patients: direct contractility (dP/dt-max) Screening when the guidelines do not apply. JACC Clin Electrophysiol 2017;3(8):830–41.
4. Cazeau S, Leclercq C, Lavergne T, et al. Effects of multisite biventricular pacing in patients with heart failure and intraventricular conduction delay. N Engl J Med 2001;344(12):873–80.
5. Chung MK, Patton KK, Lau CP, et al. 2023 HRS/ APHRS/LAHRS guideline on cardiac physiologic pacing for the avoidance and mitigation of heart failure. Heart Rhythm 2023. https://doi.org/10.1016/j. hrthm.2023.03.1538.
6. Tantengco MV, Thomas RL, Karpawich PP. Left ventricular dysfunction after long-term right ventricular apical pacing in the young. J Am Coll Cardiol 2001;37(8):2093–100.
7. Karpawich PP, Rabah R, Haas JE. Altered cardiac histology following apical right ventricular pacing in patients with congenital atrioventricular block. Pacing Clin Electrophysiol 1999;22(9):1372–7.
8. Karpawich PP, Gates J, Stokes KB. Septal His-Purkinje ventricular pacing in canines: a new endocardial electrode approach. Pacing Clin Electrophysiol 1992; 15(11 Pt 2):2011–5.
9. Gammage MD, Marsh AM. Randomized trials for selective site pacing: do we know where we are going? Pacing Clin Electrophysiol 2004;27(6 Pt 2):878–82.
10. Deshmukh P, Casavant DA, Romanyshyn M, et al. Permanent, direct His-bundle pacing: a novel approach to cardiac pacing in patients with normal His-Purkinje activation. Circulation 2000;101(8): 869–77.
11. Surkova E, Segura T, Dimopoulos K, et al. Systolic dysfunction of the subpulmonary left ventricle is associated with the severity of heart failure in patients with a systemic right ventricle. Int J Cardiol 2021;324:66–71.
12. Foster AH, Gold MR, McLaughlin JS. Acute hemodynamic effects of atrio-biventricular pacing in humans. Ann Thorac Surg 1995;59(2):294–300.
13. Rodriguez-Cruz E, Karpawich PP, Lieberman RA, et al. Biventricular pacing as alternative therapy for dilated cardiomyopathy associated with congenital heart disease. Pacing Clin Electrophysiol 2001; 24(2):235–7.
14. Lieberman R, Padeletti L, Schreuder J, et al. Ventricular pacing lead location alters systemic hemodynamics and left ventricular function in patients with and without reduced ejection fraction. J Am Coll Cardiol 2006;48(8):1634–41.
15. Karpawich PP, Mital S. Comparative left ventricular function following atrial, septal, and apical single chamber heart pacing in the young. Pacing Clin Electrophysiol 1997;20(8 Pt 1):1983–8.
16. Willemen E, Schreurs R, Huntjens PR, et al. The left and right ventricles Respond differently to variation of pacing delays in cardiac resynchronization therapy: a combined Experimental- Computational approach. Front Physiol 2019;10:17.
17. Pujol-Lopez M, Jimenez-Arjona R, Garre P, et al. Conduction system pacing vs biventricular pacing in heart failure and wide QRS patients: LEVEL-AT trial. JACC Clin Electrophysiol 2022;8(11):1431–45.
18. Mafi Rad M, Blaauw Y, Dinh T, et al. Different regions of latest electrical activation during left bundle-branch block and right ventricular pacing in cardiac resynchronization therapy patients determined by coronary venous electro-anatomic mapping. Eur J Heart Fail 2014;16(11):1214–22.
19. Elliott MK, Strocchi M, Sieniewicz BJ, et al. Biventricular endocardial pacing and left bundle branch area pacing for cardiac resynchronization: Mechanistic insights from electrocardiographic imaging, acute

hemodynamic response, and magnetic resonance imaging. Heart Rhythm 2023;20(2):207–16.

20. Borgquist R, Mortsell D, Chaudhry U, et al. Repositioning and optimization of left ventricular lead position in nonresponders to cardiac resynchronization therapy is associated with improved ejection fraction, lower NT-proBNP values, and fewer heart failure symptoms. Heart Rhythm O2 2022;3(5):457–63.

21. Marques P, Nunes-Ferreira A, Silverio Antonio P, et al. Clinical impact of MultiPoint pacing in responders to cardiac resynchronization therapy. Pacing Clin Electrophysiol 2021;44(9):1577–84.

22. Blyakhman FA, Naidich AM, Kolchanova SG, et al. Validity of ejection fraction as a measure of myocardial functional state: impact of asynchrony. Eur J Echocardiogr 2009;10(5):613–8.

23. De Pooter J, El Haddad M, Stroobandt R, et al. Accuracy of computer-calculated and manual QRS duration assessments: clinical implications to select candidates for cardiac resynchronization therapy. Int J Cardiol 2017;236:276–82.

24. Menon D, Aggarwal S, Kadiu G, et al. Assessing non-invasive studies to evaluate resynchronization pacing Effectiveness in the young. Pediatr Cardiol 2022. https://doi.org/10.1007/s00246-022-02996-9.

25. Korantzopoulos P, Zhang Z, Li G, et al. Meta-analysis of the Usefulness of change in QRS Width to predict response to cardiac resynchronization therapy. Am J Cardiol 2016;118(9):1368–73.

26. Hawkins NM, Petrie MC, MacDonald MR, et al. Selecting patients for cardiac resynchronization therapy: electrical or mechanical dyssynchrony? Eur Heart J 2006;27(11):1270–81.

27. Bristow MR, Feldman AM, Saxon LA. Heart failure management using implantable devices for ventricular resynchronization: Comparison of medical therapy, pacing, and defibrillation in chronic heart failure (COMPANION) trial. J Card Fail 2000;6(3):276–85.

28. Khairy P, van Hare GF, Balaji S, et al. PACES/HRS Expert Consensus statement on the Recognition and management of Arrhythmias in adult congenital heart disease. Heart Rhythm 2014;11(10):e1–63.

29. Chubb H, Rosenthal DN, Almond CS, et al. Impact of cardiac resynchronization therapy on heart transplant-free survival in pediatric and congenital heart disease patients. Circ Arrhythm Electrophysiol 2020;13(4):e007925.

30. Moore JP, de Groot NMS, O'Connor M, et al. Conduction system pacing versus conventional cardiac resynchronization therapy in congenital heart disease. JACC (J Am Coll Cardiol): Clinical Electrophysiology 2023;9(3):385–93.

31. Heidenreich PA, Bozkurt B, Aguilar D, et al. 2022 AHA/ACC/HFSA guideline for the management of heart failure: a Report of the American College of Cardiology/American heart association Joint Committee on clinical Practice guidelines. Circulation 2022;145(18):e895–1032.

32. Janoušek J, Gebauer RA, Abdul-Khaliq H, et al. Cardiac resynchronisation therapy in paediatric and congenital heart disease: Differential effects in various anatomical and functional substrates. Heart 2009;95(14):1165–71.

33. Chubb H, Bulic A, Mah D, et al. Impact and Modifiers of ventricular pacing in patients with single ventricle circulation. J Am Coll Cardiol 2022;80(9):902–14.

34. Stout KK, Daniels CJ, Aboulhosn JA, et al. 2018 AHA/ACC guideline for the management of adults with congenital heart disease: a Report of the American College of Cardiology/American heart association Task force on clinical Practice guidelines. Circulation 2019;139(14):e698–800.

35. Baumgartner H, De Backer J, Babu-Narayan SV, et al. 2020 ESC Guidelines for the management of adult congenital heart disease. Eur Heart J 2021;42(6):563–645.

36. Glikson M, Nielsen JC, Kronborg MB, et al. 2021 ESC Guidelines on cardiac pacing and cardiac resynchronization therapy. Europace 2022;24(1):71–164.

37. Kirk R, Dipchand AI, Rosenthal DN, et al. The International Society for heart and Lung Transplantation guidelines for the management of pediatric heart failure: Executive summary. J Heart Lung Transplant 2014;33(9):888–909.

38. Shah MJ, Silka MJ, Silva JA, et al. 2021 PACES Expert Consensus statement on the indications and management of cardiovascular implantable Electronic devices in pediatric patients. Cardiol Young 2021;1–104.

39. Epstein AE, DiMarco JP, Ellenbogen KA, et al. 2012 ACCF/AHA/HRS focused update of the 2008 guidelines for device-based therapy of cardiac Rhythm abnormalities. Circ J 2013;127:e283–352.

40. Abraham WT, Fisher WG, Smith AL, et al. Cardiac resynchronization in chronic heart failure. N Engl J Med 2002;346(24):1845–53.

41. Bristow MR, Saxon LA, Boehmer JP, et al. Cardiac resynchronization therapy with or without an implantable defibrillator in advanced chronic heart failure. N Engl J Med 2004;350:2140–50.

42. Linde C, Abraham WT, Gold MR, et al. Randomized trial of cardiac resynchronization in Mildly symptomatic heart failure patients and in Asymptomatic patients with left ventricular dysfunction and previous heart failure symptoms. J Am Coll Cardiol 2008;52(23):1834–43.

43. Moss AJ, Hall WJ, Cannom DS, et al. Cardiac-resynchronization therapy for the prevention of heart-failure Events. N Engl J Med 2009;361(12):1329–38.

44. Tang ASL, Wells GA, Talajic M, et al. Cardiac-resynchronization therapy for Mild-to-Moderate heart failure. N Engl J Med 2010;363(25):2385–95.

45. Dubin AM, Janousek J, Rhee E, et al. Resynchronization therapy in pediatric and congenital heart disease patients. J Am Coll Cardiol 2005;46(12): 2277–83.

46. Cecchin F, Frangini Pa, Brown DW, et al. Cardiac resynchronization therapy (and multisite pacing) in pediatrics and congenital heart disease: five years experience in a single institution. Journal of cardiovascular electrophysiology 2009;20(1):58–65.

47. Sakaguchi H, Miyazaki A, Yamada O, et al. Cardiac resynchronization therapy for various systemic ventricular Morphologies in patients with congenital heart disease. Circ J 2015;79(3):649–55.

48. Flugge AK, Wasmer K, Orwat S, et al. Cardiac resynchronization therapy in congenital heart disease: results from the German National Register for congenital heart defects. Int J Cardiol 2018;273: 108–11.

49. Koyak Z, de Groot JR, Krimly A, et al. Cardiac resynchronization therapy in adults with congenital heart disease. Europace 2018;20(2):315–22.

50. Leyva F, Zegard A, Qiu T, et al. Long-term outcomes of cardiac resynchronization therapy in adult congenital heart disease. Pacing Clin Electrophysiol 2019;42(6):573–80.

51. Cano O, Dandamudi G, Schaller RD, et al. Safety and feasibility of conduction system pacing in patients with congenital heart disease. J Cardiovasc Electrophysiol 2021;32(10):2692–703.

52. Chubb H, Mah D, Dubin A, et al. Conduction system pacing in pediatric and congenital heart disease. Front Physiol 2023;14. 1154629.

53. Vijayaraman P, Zalavadia D, Haseeb A, et al. Clinical outcomes of conduction system pacing compared to biventricular pacing in patients requiring cardiac resynchronization therapy. Heart Rhythm 2022; 19(8):1263–71.

54. Chung ES, Leon AR, Tavazzi L, et al. Results of the predictors of response to CRT (PROSPECT) trial. Circulation 2008;117(20):2608–16.

55. Rickard J, Michtalik H, Sharma R, et al. Predictors of response to cardiac resynchronization therapy: a systematic review. Int J Cardiol 2016;225:345–52.

56. Risum N, Jons C, Olsen NT, et al. Simple regional strain pattern analysis to predict response to cardiac resynchronization therapy: Rationale, initial results, and advantages. Am Heart J 2012;163(4):697–704.

57. Rösner A, Khalapyan T, Dalen H, et al. Classic-pattern dyssynchrony in Adolescents and adults with a Fontan circulation. J Am Soc Echocardiogr 2018;31:211–9.

58. Joyce J, O'Leary ET, Mah DY, et al. Cardiac resynchronization therapy improves the ventricular function of patients with Fontan physiology. Am Heart J 2020;230:82–92.

59. Janousek J, Kovanda J, Lozek M, et al. Pulmonary right ventricular resynchronization in congenital heart disease: acute improvement in right ventricular Mechanics and contraction Efficiency. Circ Cardiovasc Imaging 2017;10(9).

60. Thambo J-b, Guillebon MD, Xhaet O, et al. Biventricular pacing in patients with Tetralogy of Fallot : noninvasive epicardial mapping and clinical impact. Int J Cardiol 2013;163(2):170–4.

61. Janousek J, Kovanda J, Lozek M, et al. Cardiac resynchronization therapy for treatment of chronic subpulmonary right ventricular dysfunction in congenital heart disease. Circ Arrhythm Electrophysiol 2019; 12(5):e007157.

Techniques for Cardiac Resynchronization Therapy in Patients with Congenital Heart Disease

Frank J. Zimmerman, MD*, David Gamboa, MD

KEYWORDS

- Congenital heart disease • Cardiac resynchronization therapy • ECHO • RVOT
- Electroanatomic mapping • QRS

KEY POINTS

- Cardiac conduction defects and need for ventricular pacing is not uncommon with complex congenital cardiac conditions such as single ventricle physiology, systemic right ventricle and sub-pulmonic right ventricle.
- Techniques for CRT in those congenital heart disease conditions often require epicardial pacing lead placement and electroanatomic mapping for sites of delayed conduction.
- Short-term outcomes have shown favorable response for CRT in complex congenital heart disease but standardization of indications and long-term studies are needed.

INTRODUCTION

Cardiac resynchronization for congenital heart disease (CHD) has shown promising success as an adjunct to medical therapy for heart failure.[1] This is especially important for certain CHD conditions such as those with a systemic right ventricle (SRV) or single ventricle physiology in which medical therapy for heart failure has not been well established. Cardiac conduction defects are not uncommon in CHD, either as a component of the intrinsic heart disease or following surgery. Chronic ventricular pacing in certain CHD conditions can lead to detrimental effects on ventricular function, similar to those described in adults.[2,3] Collective data from existing pediatric and CHD literature show that approximately 50% of those undergoing cardiac resynchronization therapy (CRT) have had an earlier single-site ventricular pacing.[1] Although the indications, techniques, and targets for lead placement for CRT in the setting of structurally normal hearts have been well described, application of this therapy to the CHD population continues to evolve. The general principles of CRT in the structurally normal heart must be modified when applied to those with complex CHD. To "standardize" the approaches to CRT in CHD, 4 general anatomic conditions have been defined: biventricular anatomy with a systemic left ventricle, biventricular anatomy with an SRV, resynchronization of the subpulmonic right ventricle, and resynchronization for single ventricle physiology. The objective of this article is to describe the techniques used for resynchronization therapy in those patients with the following conditions: single ventricle physiology, subpulmonic right ventricle, and SRV. We will not be discussing those with biventricular anatomy with the systemic left ventricle because there is a substantial amount of literature in both the pediatric and adult populations for this condition.

CARDIAC RESYNCHRONIZATION THERAPY FOR SINGLE VENTRICLE PHYSIOLOGY

Single-site ventricular pacing in single ventricle physiology has been shown to have an adverse

Advocate Children's Heart Institute, 4440 West 95th Street, Oak Lawn, IL 60453, USA
* Corresponding author.
E-mail address: Frank.zimmerman@aah.org

Card Electrophysiol Clin 15 (2023) 447–455
https://doi.org/10.1016/j.ccep.2023.07.003
1877-9182/23/© 2023 Elsevier Inc. All rights reserved.

influence on heart function and has increased the risk for heart transplant or death. Bullock and colleagues showed progressive decline in ventricular function and subsequent development of heart failure or need for heart transplant in those with single ventricle physiology and single-site ventricular pacing.[2] In an international multicenter study, Chubb and colleagues compared single-site ventricular pacing in those with single ventricle physiology to age-matched controls.[3] They found that ventricular pacing was associated with an increased risk for heart transplant or death. The use of multisite pacing to achieve CRT in this population has been met with mixed results. One report by O'Leary and colleagues showed that CRT resulted in less of a decrease in function or need for transplant over time compared with single-site ventricular pacing.[4]

The challenges for CRT in single ventricle physiology include lack of established criteria for selection of candidates, limited access to lead placement, and lack of standardized methods to determine response to CRT. For example, the finding of a wide QRS with typical left bundle branch block (LBBB) pattern, which is a predictor of successful CRT in structurally normal hearts, is seldomly seen in those with single ventricle physiology.[5] Another challenge to CRT in single ventricle physiology is the lack of transvenous access to critical structures such as the systemic ventricle or coronary sinus. The risk of thrombus prohibits the use of transvenous leads in the systemic circulation in this population.[6] Therefore, pacing lead placement is limited to the epicardial approach, which often involves an extensive dissection and a lengthy surgery. Finally, there has been a lack of standardized methods for determination of response to CRT. This is mainly because measurement of ventricular function in complex CHD in the past has been challenging. Because earlier studies have used different definitions of CRT response, it is difficult to compare the efficacy of various lead placement strategies in this population.

Precardiac Resynchronization Therapy Assessment in Single Ventricle Physiology

Pre-CRT assessment for those with single ventricle physiology commonly involves some measurement of ventricular function. Various echocardiogram (ECHO) methods such as 3D volume, global longitudinal strain, or fractional area of shortening have been used in previous studies. Other methods of systolic performance, which are less influenced by nonstandard ventricular anatomy, include Tei index or dP/dt. For example, Karpawich and colleagues

used dP/dt response to temporary CRT to identify candidates for chronic CRT.[7]

Techniques for Cardiac Resynchronization Therapy for Single Ventricle Physiology

The most common technique described in the literature for CRT lead placement is empiric placement of pacing leads on lateral walls of the systemic ventricle as far apart as possible (**Fig. 1**A). This strategy has been described in adults with structurally normal hearts. Right ventricle (RV) and left ventricle (LV) leads are positioned distant from each other with an intrinsic delay of at least 70 milliseconds correlating with better outcomes.[8] This technique was described by Bacha and colleagues in an acute postoperative study of 26 patients with single ventricle physiology.[9] They placed temporary epicardial pacing leads on the right and left lateral ventricular walls as far apart as possible. A third lead was placed on the apex and used as the anode. The AV interval was programmed so ventricular pacing would fuse with intrinsic AV node conduction. They found that CRT resulted in an overall increase in systemic blood pressure, cardiac index, and improvement of cardiac synchronization by 3D echocardiography. Empiric placement of chronic pacing leads on the lateral walls was also described in 7 patients with single ventricle physiology in a multicenter study by Dubin and colleagues. Two of the 7 had clinical improvement, and all 7 had decreased QRS duration.[1] Finally, Karpawich and colleagues described 4 patients with single ventricle physiology that had pre-CRT screening (pacing from the lateral walls with temporary transvenous catheters and measurement of dP/dt).[7] Two of the 4 had positive responses to acute CRT (>15% increase in dP/dt) and underwent placement of chronic CRT devices using epicardial lead placement.

A second technique for CRT lead placement is to position one lead on the apex of the systemic ventricle and then to "optimize" the position of the second lead (**Fig. 1**B). The basis for this technique was described by Havalad and colleagues.[10] They performed acute CRT in the postoperative setting using 11 different temporary pacing lead configurations. They found that while there was not a single configuration that led to the best hemodynamic response, positioning one of the leads on the apex was a common denominator for the best pacing configuration in all cases. Materna and colleagues described this technique in a case report of CRT in a patient with single ventricle physiology.[11] They placed one lead on the apex of the single ventricle and then performed

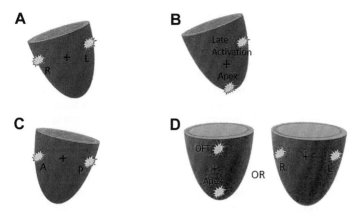

Fig. 1. Cardiac resynchronization strategies for single ventricle physiology. (*A*) Epicardial leads are empirically placed on right and left lateral walls of the single ventricle. (*B*) One epicardial lead is placed on the apex of the single ventricle and the other lead is placed at the site of latest ventricular activation determined by epicardial or intracardiac mapping. (*C*) Epicardial leads are empirically placed in an anterior and posterior position on the single ventricle. (*D*) Single right ventricle longitudinal and circumferential dyssynchrony patterns are first determined by angiography or by ECHO during sinus rhythm. In those with longitudinal dyssynchrony, the epicardial leads are placed on the RV outflow tract and RV apex. In those with circumferential dyssynchrony, the epicardial leads are placed on the right and left lateral walls of the single right ventricle. A, anterior, L, left, OFT, outflow tract, P, posterior, R, right. Yellow star, site of stimulation. Red chamber, single ventricle (right or left morphology). Blue chamber, single right ventricle.

activation mapping to identify the latest site of activation for positioning the second ventricular lead.

A third technique for CRT lead placement is to position the epicardial leads in an anterior-posterior orientation (**Fig. 1**C). In a single-center study by O'Leary and colleagues, 19 patients with single ventricle physiology underwent CRT.[4] Seven had leads placed in an anterior-posterior position while the remaining were not. There was no change in systolic ventricular function measured by 2D ECHO with CRT compared with single-site pacing. However, in a follow-up study by the same center, those with CRT were found to have improvement in dP/dt and Tei index compared with those with single-site pacing.[12]

A fourth technique for CRT lead placement in those with single ventricle physiology of RV morphology has been described by Miyazaki and colleagues (**Fig. 1**D).[13] They first determined the degree of longitudinal or circumferential dyssynchrony using angiography in 11 patients with single-RV physiology (with and without a residual LV chamber). In those with significant longitudinal dyssynchrony, placement of epicardial leads on the RV outflow tract and RV apex improved the dyssynchrony index. In those without longitudinal dyssynchrony, epicardial leads were placed on the lateral walls of the right and left ventricles. Overall, they found clinical improvement in 8 out of 11 patients undergoing chronic CRT using this strategy.

Postcardiac Resynchronization Therapy Assessment in Single Ventricle Physiology

Optimization of CRT programming in patients with single ventricle physiology has not been well described. In those with intact AV node conduction,

programming of the AV intervals to achieve the shortest QRS duration (fusion of intrinsic conduction with pacing) is commonly described. However, this strategy is limited by the fact that the degree of fusion may change with the level of activity and catecholamine state of the patient. In those patients with complete heart block, adjustment of AV interval and V-V timing can be optimized using ECHO parameters of systolic function or adjustment to achieve the shortest QRS duration. Optimization of AV and VV intervals could also be performed by assessing the degree of synchronization measured by ECHO. In a crossover trial of 14 patients with CHD, optimization by synchronization using echocardiogram was not superior to programming shortest QRS duration.[14]

CARDIAC RESYNCHRONIZATION THERAPY FOR SUBPULMONIC RIGHT VENTRICLE

RV dysfunction and RV failure are not uncommon in certain CHD conditions and can be due to several factors. A common condition associated with RV dysfunction is repaired tetralogy of Fallot. Right bundle branch block (RBBB) and RV dyssynchrony after surgery for tetralogy of Fallot have been associated with RV dilatation, reduced systolic function, and pathologic RV remodeling.[15] Hui and colleagues found that up to 93% of those with repaired tetralogy of Fallot have RV dyssynchrony and thus could be a target for resynchronization.[16] CRT for the subpulmonic RV following tetralogy of Fallot (TOF) repair was first described in acute pacing studies using temporary epicardial pacing leads.[17–19] Although those studies showed overall positive results of acute RV resynchronization, there are limited data on chronic CRT of the subpulmonic RV. Janousek and colleagues described chronic CRT for 6 patients with RBBB and subpulmonic RV dysfunction.[20] CRT resulted in improved RV dP/dt, Tei index, pulmonary artery VTI, and RV fractional area of change.

The challenges to CRT of the subpulmonic RV include lack of standard definition of response to CRT, difficulty with transvenous lead placement in nonstandard RV locations, and lack of established indications for treatment. For example, the indications for CRT with non-LBBB in adults with LV dysfunction range from Class 2A to Class 3 (depending on QRS duration) and vary between the different international society guidelines.[21,22]

Precardiac Resynchronization Therapy Assessment for the Subpulmonic Right Ventricle

Pre-CRT assessment for those with a subpulmonic ventricle includes the evaluation of RV function using ECHO, computed tomography (CT), or cardiac MRI. Assessment of RV strain or dyssynchrony is now becoming routine with advances in ECHO technology. Invasive measurement of RV dP/dt can also be performed and used to assess response to acute CRT of the subpulmonic RV.[19]

Techniques for Cardiac Resynchronization Therapy for the Subpulmonic Right Ventricle

A common technique for CRT of the subpulmonic right ventricle is empiric placement of a single lead (on the lateral RV free wall, RV apex, or RV outflow tract [RVOT]) and adjustment of the AV interval to maximize fusion with intrinsic cardiac conduction (**Fig. 2**A). This was first described by Janousek and colleagues in an acute postop study of 7 patients with CHD and RBBB.[18] They placed an epicardial temporary pacing lead on the lateral wall of the RV and performed AV sequential pacing to achieve fusion with intrinsic conduction. This resulted in the improvement in systolic blood pressure and shortening of the QRS duration. Dubin and colleagues described acute RV CRT using a single transvenous pacing lead placed empirically in the RV apex, RVOT, or RV septum.[19] They found an improvement of RV dP/dt and cardiac output with RV pacing but the optimal pacing site varied among patients. Although the optimal site did not correlate with the narrowest QRS, there was a strong relationship between the degree of QRS shortening and increase in cardiac output. Vojtovic and colleagues performed acute RV CRT in 28 postop patients with RBBB by placing a single lead on the lateral RV free wall.[23] They chose an empiric target at the border of the inflow and outflow of the RV near the TV annulus based on prior ventricular activation mapping studies of patients with RBBB. They demonstrated an increase in systolic BP, cardiac index, and LV dP/dt, which correlated with the length of time from the onset of the QRS to the local activation time of the RV lead.

A second technique for CRT of the subpulmonic right ventricle is to position a single pacing lead on the site of latest RV activation determined by intracardiac mapping (**Fig. 2**B). Janousek and colleagues described intraoperative activation mapping of the right ventricle during sinus rhythm in 6 patients with RV dysfunction and RBBB.[20] A single-RV pacing lead was then positioned at the site of latest activation and AV sequential pacing was performed. They found an improvement in RV dP/dt, Tei index, RV fractional area of change, and pulmonary artery VTI with RV CRT. Mah and colleagues described using transvenous RV activation maps obtained with a CARTO 3D catheter mapping system to locate the site of latest activation during sinus rhythm.[24] The study included 3 patients with RBBB and RV dysfunction after repair of tetralogy of Fallot. Once the RV activation maps were obtained, a chronic transvenous lead was placed in the RV apex (for sensing only) and a second lead positioned at the site of latest RV activation. CRT was performed with AV sequential pacing to achieve the shortest QRS duration. They found an improvement in RV ejection fraction in 2 out of 3 patients.

A third technique for CRT of the subpulmonic right ventricle is to perform active pacing from 2 sites in right ventricle (**Fig. 2**C). This was first described in an acute postoperative study of 10 patients with CHD and RBBB.[17] Temporary epicardial pacing leads were positioned on the RVOT and lateral RV free wall. A third lead was placed on the apex for the anode. Multisite pacing from the RVOT and RV lateral wall resulted in an improvement of systolic BP and cardiac index. Multisite RV pacing was also described in a case report by Markel and colleagues in a patient with repaired tetralogy of Fallot and LV dysfunction.[25] They placed permanent transvenous pacing leads in the RV apex and RV free wall. AV sequential pacing using the 2 RV leads resulted in a decrease in QRS duration and an improvement of LV function.

A fourth technique for CRT of the subpulmonic right ventricle is to perform standard biventricular CRT using one lead in RV and a second lead in coronary sinus for LV pacing (**Fig. 2**D). This was first described by Thambo and colleagues in 8 patients with repaired tetralogy of Fallot and severe RV dysfunction.[26] The mean left ventricular ejection fraction (LVEF) for this group was 56.2 ± 10.1% before pacing. Acute biventricular CRT resulted in

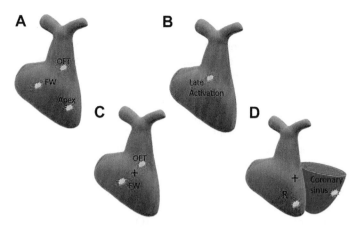

Fig. 2. Cardiac resynchronization strategies for subpulmonary right ventricle. (*A*) Single epicardial or transvenous lead can be placed empirically on the RV apex, RV outflow tract, or RV free wall. (*B*) Single epicardial or transvenous lead can be placed at the site of latest ventricular activation determined by intracardiac or epicardial mapping. (*C*) Epicardial or transvenous leads can be placed on the RV free wall and RV outflow tract and simultaneous pacing from both sites can be performed. (*D*) Transvenous lead placed in RV apex and left ventricular lead placed via coronary sinus. Simultaneous pacing is then performed from both sites to achieve CRT. FW, free wall, OFT, outflow tract, R, right. Yellow star, site of stimulation. Blue chamber, subpulmonic right ventricle. Red chamber, subaortic left ventricle.

a decrease in QRS duration and an acute improvement in RV and LV dP/dt. Thambo and colleagues also evaluated the effects of chronic biventricular pacing in 9 patients with repaired tetralogy of Fallot.[27] They found an improvement of global activation and electrical dyssynchrony index compared with sinus rhythm and single-site RV pacing. They also found an improvement of New York Heart Association (NYHA) class, exercise test performance, and LVEF (50 ± 8% to 56 ± 8%) with biventricular pacing compared with baseline.

Postcardiac Resynchronization Therapy Assessment for the Subpulmonic Right Ventricle

Optimization of CRT for the subpulmonic RV consists mainly of adjusting AV intervals to maximize fusion with intrinsic conduction achieving the shortest QRS duration. The limitation with this technique is that AV conduction and maximal fusion will vary depending on the activity level of the patient and possibly RV lead location.[28] This is less of an issue with multisite RV or biventricular pacing. Assessment of RV response to CRT can be performed using standard echocardiography, strain imaging, or cardiac CT/MRI. Assessment of functional status using cardiopulmonary stress testing before and after CRT may be useful for this population but has not been consistently reported in prior studies.[27]

CARDIAC RESYNCHRONIZATION THERAPY FOR THE SYSTEMIC RIGHT VENTRICLE

An SRV is encountered either in patients with congenitally corrected transposition of the great arteries (CCTGA) or in patients with dextrotransposition of the great arteries (DTGA) with previous atrial switch repair (Mustard or Senning). Development of heart failure is frequent in this population: by age 45 years, up to 65% of patients with an SRV have symptomatic heart failure.[29] The role for CRT was suggested in a study by Jauvert and colleagues demonstrating that ventricular dysfunction was in part due to electromechanical dyssynchrony.[30] In a study of 120 patients, established indications for CRT (NYHA class >2, QRS duration >120 milliseconds) were found in 9.3% of those with DTGA s/p atrial switch and 6.1% of those with CCTGA.[31] In a multicenter study by Dubin and colleagues, 13 out of 17 patients with SRV had an improvement of RV ejection fraction with CRT.[1] In another multicenter study by Janousek and colleagues, 24 out of 27 patients with SRV had an improvement of RV ejection fraction with CRT.[32] However, the degree of AV valve regurgitation remained higher in those with an SRV compared with those with systemic LV after CRT.

The challenges for CRT in this population include the fact that the access to critical structures such as the coronary sinus is often not possible. Placement of an epicardial pacing lead is often required in order to achieve CRT. There are no consensus guidelines for optimal lead position or indications for CRT in those with an SRV. Finally, earlier studies have used a variety of methods to assess systemic RV function after CRT, making it difficult to compare different pacing strategies in this population.

Precardiac Resynchronization Therapy Assessment for the Systemic RV

Patients with an SRV require special considerations when planning a procedure for CRT. Coronary sinus abnormalities are common in patients with CCTGA.[33] In patients with DTGA s/p atrial switch, the coronary sinus may not be accessible from the systemic venous atrial side.[34] The use of preprocedural imaging in patients with DTGA s/p atrial switch or with CCTGA has been recognized as a useful adjunct for planning CRT implantation.[35] A retrospective review of 7 patients with CCTGA or DTGA s/p Mustard or Senning described the benefit of advanced imaging for planning of the procedure. Three patients underwent cardiac CT, and 4 underwent coronary angiography with levophase imaging of the coronary sinus (CS) or direct contrast injection of the CS. Based on the findings of the coronary venous anatomy, 3 patients required surgical placement of a lead, whereas 4 were able to undergo transvenous placement.

Techniques for Cardiac Resynchronization Therapy for the Systemic Right Ventricle

One technique of CRT with SRV is to place one pacing lead on the morphologic LV (subpulmonic ventricle), either transvenous or epicardial, and then to place a second ventricular pacing lead laterally on the epicardial surface of the systemic RV (subaortic ventricle) (**Fig. 3**A). This technique was described in 8 patients (4 with DTGA s/p atrial switch) with SRV and reduced RV systolic function.[36] The RV leads were placed on areas of late activation by measuring local activation times (LATs) from the epicardium. CRT resulted in midterm improvement in RV function, RV dP/dt, and NYHA functional classification. However, the

degree of tricuspid valve regurgitation was not significantly influenced by CRT.

Placement of the epicardial RV lead in those with SRV can also be guided by electroanatomic mapping to identify the site of latest activation during sinus rhythm (**Fig. 3**B). This technique was described by Moore and colleagues and involves a hybrid approach to CRT placement.[37] Six patients (3 with CCTGA and 3 with DTGA and Mustard or Senning) who had a preexisting transvenous dual-chamber pacemaker or implantable cardioverter defibrillator (ICD) were taken to the hybrid laboratory for the 2-step procedure. First electroanatomic mapping (EAM) was performed using CARTO while in the patient's baseline rhythm (DDD pacing for those with underlying complete AV block and AAI pacing for those with intact AV conduction). Access to the SRV was achieved using retrograde arterial approach. LATs were recorded within the entire RV endocardial surface. Following the mapping procedure, the catheter was placed at the site of latest activation, and biplane cine fluoroscopy was used to record its location. Then an incision was made (limited left thoracotomy in cases of CCTGA; lower midsternotomy for DTGA after Mustard or Senning) and epicardial mapping of the RV region across from the previously identified endocardial target for the latest epicardial activation was performed. The latest activation occurred at the basolateral RV, just apical to the tricuspid valve annulus. The superior-inferior position was the most variable feature of endocardial activation: for patients with intact AV conduction,

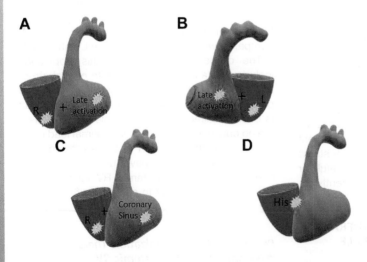

Fig. 3. Cardiac resynchronization strategies for systemic right ventricle. (*A*) Lead placement for CCTGA. One transvenous lead is placed in the apex of the right-sided subpulmonic ventricle (morphologic left ventricle). Second epicardial lead is placed on the systemic right ventricle at the site of latest ventricular activation determined by intracardiac or epicardial mapping. (*B*) Lead placement for DTGA s/p atrial switch. One transvenous lead is placed in the apex of the subpulmonic ventricle (morphologic left ventricle). A second epicardial lead is placed either empirically or at the site of latest ventricular activation on the systemic right ventricle. (*C*) Lead placement for CCTGA. One transvenous lead is placed in the apex of the subpulmonic ventricle (morphologic left ventricle). A second transvenous lead is placed in the systemic RV via the coronary sinus. (*D*) Lead placement for CCTGA. A single transvenous lead is placed in the subpulmonic ventricle (morphologic left ventricle) at site of His for conduction-system pacing. L, left, R, right. Yellow star, site of stimulation. Blue chamber, systemic right ventricle. Red chamber, subpulmonic left ventricle.

the latest activation was localized to sites around the inferior-to-midportion of the tricuspid valve annulus and for patients with chronic ventricular pacing, the latest activation was located at more superior sites and often involved the inferior portion of the RV outflow tract. CRT using this technique resulted in favorable outcomes: the median QRS duration decreased from 193 to 147 milliseconds ($P < .001$), and NYHA functional class decreased in all patients (including resolution of symptoms in 3 patients). There was a quantitative improvement in echocardiographic RV systolic function in 5 patients, with a median increase in RV fractional area of change from 15.5% to 30% for all patients following CRT ($P < .001$).

A totally transvenous CRT implantation technique was described by Moore and colleagues in 20 patients with CCTGA (**Fig. 3**C).[38] Indications for CRT were classified as (1) congestive heart failure with intact AV conduction and QRS prolongation, (2) cardiomyopathy related to chronic LV pacing, or (3) complete AV block with anticipation of more than 40% ventricular pacing. In the early years, there was selective coronary angiography during implantation to evaluate coronary venous drainage. In later years, preprocedure CT angiography was performed to delineate the coronary venous anatomy. After selective coronary angiography with levophase filling of the coronary venous anatomy, access to the subclavian vein was obtained, the CS ostium was cannulated with a luminal decapolar catheter, and a sheath advanced into the CS. For patients without conventional coronary venous drainage, access to the ectopic coronary ostium was obtained with the use of a variety of preformed catheters and guidewires, and the delivery sheath and dilater were advanced over the wire and into the ectopic vein. Once venous access was obtained, wedge venography was performed to outline the anatomy in its entirety. Coronary venous drainage was classified as (1) conventional, (2) dual ostia, (3) separate ostia, and (4) vein of Marshall-dependent. Final lead position was classified as within the RV body versus RVOT. There was procedural success in 18 out of 19 patients who underwent attempted transvenous CRT lead placement. Despite variability in anatomic origins, a postero-septal CS ostium was used for lead delivery in 14 of 18 leads. Two patients with separate ostia underwent cannulation of a superior CS ostium, and 2 patients with vein of Marshall-dependent anatomy underwent placement of lead from the innominate vein. The final lead position was within the RV body in 12 (60%) patients and RVOT in 8 (40%). After CRT, the median QRS duration decreased by 18 milliseconds (interquartile range [IQR]: 38–14 milliseconds). Of the 12 patients with NYHA class 2 or greater at the time of CRT, 8 (67%) had a positive response. Location of the CS lead in the RVOT was the only predictor of poor outcome among covariates tested, possibly because the RV relies more on circumferential shortening rather than longitudinal shortening in the setting of chronic pressure overload.[39]

Finally, transvenous conduction system pacing can be used as a method for CRT in patients with CCTGA (**Fig. 3**D). Moore and colleagues described this technique in 15 patients with CCTGA undergoing CRT.[40] Conduction system pacing was successful in 13 out of 15 patients (His bundle in 11, LBB pacing in 2). CRT resulted in decrease in QRS duration in those who had earlier conventional pacing, and NYHA functional class improved in 5 patients. However, qualitative RV systolic function did not improve after median follow-up of 8 months.

Postcardiac Resynchronization Therapy Assessment

There are no standard criteria for evaluating response to CRT in patients with SRV. The quantification of systolic function of the right ventricle has presented challenges due to reliability of measurements using echocardiogram. Exercise parameters such as peak oxygen consumption (peak V_{O_2}) and peak heart rate may be useful for a standard assessment of CRT response in this population.[41]

SUMMARY

CRT for complex CHD has shown favorable results and may serve as an important adjunct to medical therapy for the failing systemic or subpulmonary ventricle. However, CRT for this population is complicated and often requires the need for placement of epicardial pacing leads or extensive periprocedure ventricular activation mapping. Preprocedure and postprocedure assessments often involve some measurement of ventricular function or synchrony, which can be challenging due to the lack of standardization of these methods in complex CHD.

CLINICS CARE POINTS

- Chronic ventricular pacing for those with single ventricle physiology is associated with an increased risk for heart transplant or death.

- Multisite ventricular pacing in this population can result in an acute clinical improvement but no long-term studies are available to assess morbidity and mortality.
- Right ventricular dysfunction is not uncommon in certain congenital heart conditions such as tetralogy of Fallot s/p repair, D-transposition of the great arteries (D-TGA) s/p atrial switch operation and L-transposition of the great arteries (L-TGA).
- Dyssynchrony of the failing right ventricle has been described and often correlates with a wide QRS.
- Resynchronization of the failing right ventricle involving different techniques than the standard biventricular pacing used in structurally normal hearts has resulted in acute clinical improvement but long-term studies are not yet available to assess the efficacy of this approach.

REFERENCES

1. Dubin AM, Janousek J, Rhee E, et al. Resynchronization therapy in pediatric and congenital heart disease patients: an international multicenter study. J Am Coll Cardiol 2005;46(12):2277–83.
2. Bulic A, Zimmerman FJ, Ceresnak SR, et al. Ventricular pacing in single ventricles-A bad combination. Heart Rhythm 2017;14(6):853–7.
3. Chubb H, Bulic A, Mah D, et al. Impact and modifiers of ventricular pacing in patients with single ventricle circulation. J Am Coll Cardiol 2022;80(9):902–14.
4. O'Leary ET, Gauvreau K, Alexander ME, et al. Dual-site ventricular pacing in patients with fontan physiology and heart block: does it mitigate the detrimental effects of single-site ventricular pacing? JACC Clin Electrophysiol 2018;4(10):1289–97.
5. Karikari Y, Abdulkarim M, Li Y, et al. The progress and significance of QRS duration by electrocardiography in hypoplastic left heart syndrome. Pediatr Cardiol 2020;41(1):141–8.
6. Khairy P, Landzberg MJ, Gatzoulis MA, et al. Transvenous pacing leads and systemic thromboemboli in patients with intracardiac shunts: a multicenter study. Circulation 2006;113(20):2391–7.
7. Karpawich PP, Bansal N, Samuel S, et al. 16 Years of cardiac resynchronization pacing among congenital heart disease patients: direct contractility (dP/dt-max) screening when the guidelines do not apply. JACC Clin Electrophysiol 2017;3(8):830–41.
8. Gold MR, Singh JP, Ellenbogen KA, et al. Interventricular electrical delay is predictive of response to cardiac resynchronization therapy. JACC Clin Electrophysiol 2016;2(4):438–47.
9. Bacha EA, Zimmerman FJ, Mor-Avi V, et al. Ventricular resynchronization by multisite pacing improves myocardial performance in the postoperative single-ventricle patient. Ann Thorac Surg 2004;78(5):1678–83.
10. Havalad V, Cabreriza SE, Cheung EW, et al. Optimized multisite pacing in postoperative single-ventricle patients. Pediatr Cardiol 2014;35(7):1213–9.
11. Materna O, Kubus P, Janousek J. Right ventricular resynchronization in a child with hypoplastic left heart syndrome. Heart Rhythm 2014;11(12):2303–5.
12. Joyce J, O'Leary ET, Mah DY, et al. Cardiac resynchronization therapy improves the ventricular function of patients with Fontan physiology. Am Heart J 2020;230:82–92.
13. Miyazaki A, Sakaguchi H, Kagisaki K, et al. Optimal pacing sites for cardiac resynchronization therapy for patients with a systemic right ventricle with or without a rudimentary left ventricle. Europace 2016;18(1):100–12.
14. Punn R, Hanisch D, Motonaga KS, et al. A pilot study assessing ECG versus ECHO ventriculoventricular optimization in pediatric resynchronization patients. J Cardiovasc Electrophysiol 2016;27(2):210–6.
15. Yim D, Hui W, Larios G, et al. Quantification of right ventricular electromechanical dyssynchrony in relation to right ventricular function and clinical outcomes in children with repaired tetralogy of fallot. J Am Soc Echocardiogr 2018;31(7):822–30.
16. Hui W, Slorach C, Dragulescu A, et al. Mechanisms of right ventricular electromechanical dyssynchrony and mechanical inefficiency in children after repair of tetralogy of fallot. Circ Cardiovasc Imaging 2014;7(4):610–8.
17. Zimmerman FJ, Starr JP, Koenig PR, et al. Acute hemodynamic benefit of multisite ventricular pacing after congenital heart surgery. Ann Thorac Surg 2003;75(6):1775–80.
18. Janousek J, Vojtovic P, Hucín B, et al. Resynchronization pacing is a useful adjunct to the management of acute heart failure after surgery for congenital heart defects. Am J Cardiol 2001;88(2):145–52.
19. Dubin AM, Feinstein JA, Reddy VM, et al. Electrical resynchronization: a novel therapy for the failing right ventricle. Circulation 2003;107(18):2287–9.
20. Janousek J, Kovanda J, Ložek M, et al. Cardiac resynchronization therapy for treatment of chronic subpulmonary right ventricular dysfunction in congenital heart disease. Circ Arrhythm Electrophysiol 2019;12(5):e007157.
21. Epstein AE, Dimarco JP, Ellenbogen KA, et al. ACC/AHA/HRS 2008 guidelines for device-based therapy of cardiac rhythm abnormalities: a report of the American college of cardiology/American heart association task force on practice guidelines (writing committee to revise the ACC/AHA/NASPE 2002

guideline update for implantation of cardiac pace-makers and antiarrhythmia devices) developed in collaboration with the American association for thoracic surgery and society of thoracic surgeons. J Am Coll Cardiol 2008;51(21):e1–62.

22. Brignole M, Auricchio A, Baron-Esquivias G, et al. 2013 ESC Guidelines on cardiac pacing and cardiac resynchronization therapy: the Task Force on cardiac pacing and resynchronization therapy of the European Society of Cardiology (ESC). Developed in collaboration with the European Heart Rhythm Association (EHRA). Eur Heart J 2013; 34(29):2281–329.

23. Vojtovic P, Kucera F, Kubuš P, et al. Acute right ventricular resynchronization improves haemodynamics in children after surgical repair of tetralogy of Fallot. Europace 2018;20(2):323–8.

24. Mah DY, O'Leary ET, Harrild DM, et al. Resynchronizing right and left ventricles with right bundle branch block in the congenital heart disease population. JACC Clin Electrophysiol 2020;6(14):1762–72.

25. Markel F, Paech C, Gebauer RA. Is right ventricular resynchronization the key to both right and left ventricular remodeling? HeartRhythm Case Rep 2020; 6(1):20–2.

26. Thambo JB, Dos Santos P, De Guillebon M, et al. Biventricular stimulation improves right and left ventricular function after tetralogy of Fallot repair: acute animal and clinical studies. Heart Rhythm 2010;7(3):344–50.

27. Thambo JB, De Guillebon M, Xhaet O, et al. Biventricular pacing in patients with Tetralogy of Fallot: non-invasive epicardial mapping and clinical impact. Int J Cardiol 2013;163(2):170–4.

28. Stephenson EA, Cecchin F, Alexander ME, et al. Relation of right ventricular pacing in tetralogy of Fallot to electrical resynchronization. Am J Cardiol 2004;93(11):1449–52.

29. Piran S, Veldtman G, Siu S, et al. Heart failure and ventricular dysfunction in patients with single or systemic right ventricles. Circulation 2002;105(10): 1189–94.

30. Jauvert G, Rousseau-Paziaud J, Villain E, et al. Effects of cardiac resynchronization therapy on echocardiographic indices, functional capacity, and clinical outcomes of patients with a systemic right ventricle. Europace 2009;11(2):184–90.

31. Diller GP, Okonko D, Uebing A, et al. Cardiac resynchronization therapy for adult congenital heart disease patients with a systemic right ventricle: analysis of feasibility and review of early experience. Europace 2006;8(4):267–72.

32. Janousek J, Gebauer RA, Abdul-Khaliq H, et al. Cardiac resynchronisation therapy in paediatric and congenital heart disease: differential effects in various anatomical and functional substrates. Heart 2009;95(14):1165–71.

33. Bottega NA, Kapa S, Edwards WD, et al. The cardiac veins in congenitally corrected transposition of the great arteries: delivery options for cardiac devices. Heart Rhythm 2009;6(10):1450–6.

34. Ebert PA, Gay WA Jr, Engle MA. Correction of transposition of the great arteries: relationship of the coronary sinus and postoperative arrhythmias. Ann Surg 1974;180(4):433–8.

35. Ruckdeschel ES, Quaife R, Lewkowiez L, et al. Preprocedural imaging in patients with transposition of the great arteries facilitates placement of cardiac resynchronization therapy leads. Pacing Clin Electrophysiol 2014;37(5):546–53.

36. Janousek J, Tomek V, Chaloupecký VA, et al. Cardiac resynchronization therapy: a novel adjunct to the treatment and prevention of systemic right ventricular failure. J Am Coll Cardiol 2004;44(9): 1927–31.

37. Moore JP, Gallotti RG, Shannon KM, et al. A minimally invasive hybrid approach for cardiac resynchronization of the systemic right ventricle. Pacing Clin Electrophysiol 2019;42(2):171–7.

38. Moore JP, Cho D, Lin JP, et al. Implantation techniques and outcomes after cardiac resynchronization therapy for congenitally corrected transposition of the great arteries. Heart Rhythm 2018;15(12):1808–15.

39. Pettersen E, Helle-Valle T, Edvardsen T, et al. Contraction pattern of the systemic right ventricle shift from longitudinal to circumferential shortening and absent global ventricular torsion. J Am Coll Cardiol 2007;49(25):2450–6.

40. Moore JP, Gallotti R, Shannon KM, et al. Permanent conduction system pacing for congenitally corrected transposition of the great arteries: a pediatric and congenital electrophysiology society (PACES)/ International society for adult congenital heart disease (ISACHD) collaborative study. Heart Rhythm 2020;S1547-5271(20):30088–96.

41. Diller GP, Dimopoulos K, Okonko D, et al. Exercise intolerance in adult congenital heart disease. Circulation 2005;112:828–35.

Conduction System Pacing for Patients with Congenital Heart Disease

Jeremy P. Moore, MD, MS[a,b,c],*, Aarti S. Dalal, DO[d]

KEYWORDS

- Conduction system pacing • Physiologic pacing • Cardiac resynchronization therapy
- Electromechanical dyssynchrony • His bundle pacing • Left bundle branch area pacing

KEY POINTS

- Conduction system pacing (CSP) techniques have been applied to patients with biventricular congenital heart disease (CHD), both with systemic left and right ventricular anatomical morphologies.
- CSP may prevent or reverse the adverse consequences of electromechanical dyssynchrony for a wide variety of CHD.
- For patients with biventricular CHD characterized by a systemic left ventricle (LV), CSP seems at least equivalent to conventional cardiac resynchronization therapy for LV remodeling.
- Further study of the merits of CSP in CHD is recommended.

INTRODUCTION

Over the past decade, conduction system pacing (CSP) has emerged not only as a viable, but many times the preferred, management option for permanent cardiac pacing among patients for whom there is concern for electromechanical dyssynchrony. An increasingly sophisticated understanding of conduction system physiology, improved technical skills, and the rapid expansion of dedicated tools has permitted the widespread adoption of this approach.

Although previously applied to patients with structurally normal hearts with acquired forms of heart disease, patients affected by congenital heart disease (CHD) also stand to benefit from this innovative approach. Patients with CHD are particularly vulnerable to the adverse effects of permanent ventricular pacing that is often used relatively early in life. Recent studies have demonstrated that CSP is not only feasible and safe in the population with CHD, but it is associated with clinically relevant functional improvement that is on par with that observed after conventional cardiac resynchronization therapy (CRT).

The following text aims to summarize existing knowledge surrounding CSP in CHD with a special emphasis on the unique opportunities and challenges in this population. CHDs are grouped according to the dominant ventricular morphologic categories of "systemic left" and "systemic right" ventricles, given their relation to conduction system anatomy and fundamental CSP approach.

[a] Division of Cardiology, Department of Medicine, University of California Los Angeles (UCLA) Medical Center, Ahmanson/UCLA Adult Congenital Heart Disease Center, Los Angeles, CA, USA; [b] UCLA Cardiac Arrhythmia Center, UCLA Health System, David Geffen School of Medicine at UCLA, Los Angeles, CA, USA; [c] Division of Cardiology, Department of Pediatrics, UCLA Medical Center, Los Angeles, CA, USA; [d] Division of Cardiology, Monroe Carell Jr Children's Hospital, Vanderbilt University, 2200 Children's Way, Suite 5230, Nashville, TN 37232, USA
* Corresponding author. 200 Medical Plaza Drive Suite 330, Los Angeles, CA 90095.
E-mail address: jpmoore@mednet.ucla.edu

Card Electrophysiol Clin 15 (2023) 457–466
https://doi.org/10.1016/j.ccep.2023.06.009
1877-9182/23/Published by Elsevier Inc.

RATIONALE FOR CONDUCTION SYSTEM PACING IN CONGENITAL HEART DISEASE

Congenital Heart Disease with Systemic Left Ventricle Morphology

For children and adults with CHD, the most common anatomical arrangement consists of balanced ventricles with the morphologic left ventricle (LV) functioning as the subaortic pump. For such patients, the pursuit of CSP is often motivated by preexisting, or concern about future, ventricular dysfunction related to electromechanical dyssynchrony. Often, prior permanent right ventricular (RV) apical pacing has culminated in LV systolic dysfunction that may be improved by a strategy of physiologic pacing.[1]

Permanent RV pacing with resultant pacing-induced cardiomyopathy is increasingly recognized in CHD. The cumulative effects of preoperative hypoxemia, cardiac bypass surgery, and residual hemodynamic impairment create an environment in which the ventricular myocardium is poorly suited to endure years of electromechanical dyssynchrony. Estimates for pacing-induced cardiomyopathy among children and young adults with CHD range from 10% to 50% depending on the anatomic lesion, lead location, and ventricular pacing burden.[2] In this context, CSP represents an opportunity to circumvent this negative outcome by preemptive optimization of electromechanical synchrony. Alternatively, CSP can be pursued after pacing-induced cardiomyopathy has already become established in an effort to reverse this process. Finally (and less established for CHD), among patients with bundle branch block and electromechanical dyssynchrony, CSP has been used to recruit predetermined His–Purkinje fibers or directly capture the conduction system distal to the level of bundle branch block to reestablish physiologic conduction.[3]

A related strategy for physiologic pacing among CHD involves targeted septal pacing with acute hemodynamic feedback as a guide for optimal lead implant sites.[4] Although preferable to conventional apical pacing, such a strategy can yield inconsistent results and has not been reproduced in randomized trials.[5] For many patients with CHD, the initial pursuit of CSP therefore represents an opportunity to avoid the adverse consequences of permanent RV pacing. CSP may also be preferable to prophylactic conventional CRT with biventricular pacing in smaller patients with CHD to minimize intravascular lead material or prevent repeat sternotomy for the addition of an epicardial LV lead.

Congenital Heart Disease with Systemic Right Ventricular Morphology

Less common, but of considerable importance, are CHD patients born with 2 balanced ventricular chambers, but where the morphologic RV is in the subaortic position. Although several anatomical variants exist, the most common are the d-transposition of the great arteries after operations for physiologic repair (ie, Mustard or Senning operations) and those with congenitally corrected transposition of the great arteries (CCTGA). In both situations, an ill-equipped morphologic RV serves as the systemic pumping chamber.

Patients born with CCTGA are particularly vulnerable to adverse electromechanical effects of permanent ventricular pacing. Compounded by a 2% annualized risk of spontaneous AV block that prompts chronic LV pacing, a rapid decline in ventricular systolic function is observed in this group.[6,7] Likewise, patients after Mustard and Senning operations are at greater risk for deterioration in RV function with age. With the development of AV block and the initiation of permanent ventricular pacing, a precipitous decline in cardiac function is often observed. CRT with biventricular pacing is inherently challenging in this latter group, usually requiring a limited surgical lower sternotomy for access to the RV epicardium.[8]

Importantly, for both forms of CHD, the goal of CSP is to provide rapid and synchronous activation of the systemic morphologic RV following lead placement in the LV. Therefore, pacing the conduction system as proximal as possible (ie, engaging the non-branching His bundle or proximal left bundle branches) is desirable and is considered the goal of the CSP procedure. Although RV septal myocardial pacing or even direct engagement of the right bundle is theoretically possible, to date these strategies have not been well studied.

ANATOMICAL CONSIDERATIONS

In-depth knowledge of the conduction system anatomy in CHD is available from comprehensive histopathological studies. An exhaustive description of the anatomical course of the conduction system in complex CHD is beyond the scope of the review, but interested readers are encouraged to consult authoritative texts dealing with this subject.[9] The following sections will instead attempt to summarize the common conduction system variants most likely to be encountered during CSP.

Congenital Heart Disease with Systemic Left Ventricular Morphology

For most forms of CHD, only minor deviation of the AV conduction system occurs as it passes in relation to the central fibrous body near the crux of the heart. Normally, the His bundle courses briefly in a leftward and inferior relation to the membranous septum before branching broadly along the leftward aspect of the ventricular septum. The right bundle branch continues as a chord-like structure toward the rightward aspect of the ventricular septum, running through the moderator band to reach the anterolateral RV free wall before ramification.

Among patients with CHD, the essential posteroinferior relationship between the non-branching His bundle and the membranous septum is maintained, such that a negligible anatomical impact on CSP targets is expected. On the other hand, cardiac repair for common CHDs such as ventricular septal defects (VSD) can directly injure or result in postoperative scarring that jeopardizes regions surrounding the conducting tissues. Accordingly, low voltage areas and scar may be more frequently encountered when attempting his bundle pacing (HBP) in CHD patients with prior VSD closure and can negatively impact lead performance.

A separate anatomical challenge encountered among CHD is the often greatly enlarged right-sided structures owing to the effects of chronic pulmonary or tricuspid valve regurgitation. Such enlargement may impact CSP by increasing the range required to achieve left bundle branch area pacing (LBBAP). Sufficient distance to cross the AV valve annulus may be challenging despite an array of implantation tools. Additionally, the cardiac rotation that accompanies RV volume overload may distort anatomic landmarks, necessitating cautious implantation of CSP with frequent alternative fluoroscopic views for proper placement (**Fig. 1**).

Congenital Heart Disease with Systemic Right Ventricular Morphology

The conduction system anatomy associated with CCTGA has been of great interest to pathologists and was ultimately clarified after detailed histologic evaluation. In most cases, the non-branching atrioventricular (AV) bundle takes origin from an anterior AV node at the pulmonary-mitral valve continuity, from where it descends onto the ventricular septum after passing through the subpulmonary myocardium. This anomalous course places the septal non-branching His bundle in a more apical position when compared with the normal heart, which may favorably impact CSP performance. In fact, the septal conduction system is separate from the fibrous annulus and wholly contained in the working ventricular myocardium, circumventing some of the troublesome issues that accompany HBP in the general population (namely poor sensing and pacing characteristics).

Less commonly, in a subset of patients with CCTGA with favorable alignment between the inter-atrial and ventricular septae, a sling of conduction tissue may exist. For these patients, the anterior and posterior AV bundles may separately contribute to the conduction sling. This may result in a typical basal location of the posterior left bundle closer to the fibrous annulus (**Fig. 2**). Although this has not to our knowledge been formally described, this basal location for the left posterior fascicle in CCTGA is entirely consistent with original histologic descriptions of conduction sling branching.[9]

DEFINITIONS

Verification of CSP relies on specific, but evolving, criteria based on the 12 lead ECG, intracardiac electrograms, and understanding of the normal physiology of ventricular activation. Such criteria have been successfully adapted to patients with CHD despite limitations that are related to variations in ventricular situs, morphology, and position. Separate criteria for both HBP and LBBAP are described in the following text.

His Bundle Pacing Criteria

Typical criteria for selective HBP include an expected HV interval at the lead fixation site that measures greater than or equal to 35 ms with a discrete, non-captured ventricular electrogram on the unipolar recording and subsequent stimulation to QRS onset interval equal to the HV interval. The QRS morphology in this situation is expected to be nearly identical to the underlying intrinsic QRS complex. Nonselective HBP is identified when the HV interval is greater than the stimulus to QRS onset interval and a pseudo-delta wave is noted with local ventricular capture, often associated with output-dependent changes in QRS morphology.[10]

For patients with CCTGA, either HBP or proximal LBBP may be achieved and are believed to be equivalent in terms of cardiac resynchronization. For proximal left bundle branch capture, similar criteria to HBP are used, but an LBB-V interval less than or equal to 35 ms and a change in the QRS axis during pacing (relative to the native QRS) are typically observed (**Fig. 3**).

Left Bundle Branch Area Pacing Criteria

With lead fixation at the LV septum ("left bundle area pacing"), pacing capture of the left bundle branches, isolated ventricular myocardium, or both is possible. Each of these is associated with a unique electrocardiographic signature that serves as a basis for the determination of CSP. With direct capture of the left bundle branches, a

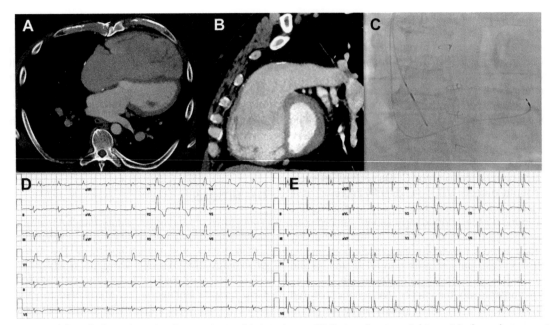

Fig. 1. Left bundle branch pacing in a patient with tetralogy of Fallot and severe right ventricular enlargement related to chronic pulmonary regurgitation. Representative (*A*) axial and (*B*) sagittal cuts of a preoperative computed tomographic scan show the dilated and posteriorly rotated ventricles and ventricular septum for a patient with tetralogy of Fallot and severe pulmonary regurgitation affected by intermittent atrioventricular block. (*C*) Anteroposterior fluoroscopic view shows greater than usual posterior lead positioning for left bundle branch pacing that had required a modified implant approach. (*D*) Intrinsic rhythm and (*E*) left bundle branch pacing QRS morphology are shown.

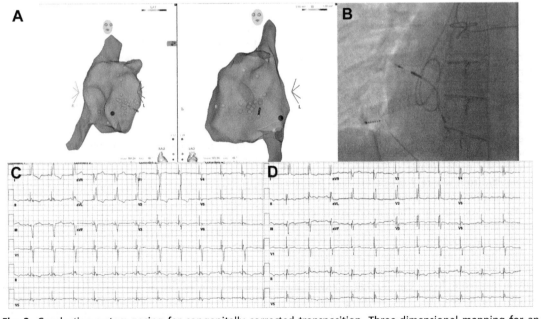

Fig. 2. Conduction system pacing for congenitally corrected transposition. Three-dimensional mapping for an adult patient with congenitally corrected transposition was performed to delineate the course of the His bundle and bundle branches. (*A*) Yellow circles indicate the location of a posteriorly situated His bundle and proximal left posterior fascicle. The lead was affixed to an inferior location where a His bundle electrogram and HV interval measuring 35 ms were observed. (*B*) The posterior (inferior) fluoroscopic lead location is shown. (*C*) and (*D*) Baseline left ventricular apical pacing and His bundle pacing, respectively.

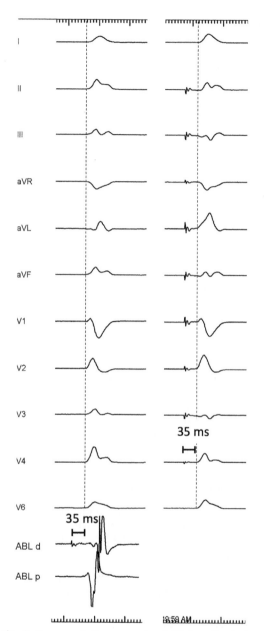

Fig. 3. Representative example of His bundle pacing for congenitally corrected transposition. The identical patient from **Fig. 2** is shown. With the lead located as depicted previously, an HV interval of 35 ms was noted, consistent with positioning at the proximal left bundle branch. In the rightward panel, pacing from this location resulted in selective left bundle pacing with isoelectric stimulus to QRS interval equal to the HV interval and minimal change in the QRS morphology.

qR or rSR pattern in V1 is observed in nearly all cases (vs approximately 25% for LV septal myocardial-only capture) and a terminal S wave in V1 is typically absent. Further confirmatory

ECG evidence of left bundle branch capture includes an LV activation time (LVAT) of less than 75 ms (interval from the stimulus artifact to the peak of the R wave in V5 or V6), reflecting rapid activation of the LV free wall, abrupt shortening of the LVAT as the lead is progressively advanced into the ventricular septum, fixation beats and a V6–V1 interpeak interval greater than 44 ms (**Fig. 4**).[11,12] Although the demonstration of a LBB potential is considered ideal, it is neither sufficient nor necessary for the demonstration of LBB pacing capture. More recently, physiology-based criteria have been proposed to enhance the confirmation of left bundle branch capture.[13]

IMPLANT TECHNIQUE

There is no universally accepted technique for the implantation of CSP leads in CHD. Nevertheless, common scenarios exist for which various solutions have been proposed. The preoperative evaluation consists of a careful review of the patient's anatomic and surgical history with an appraisal of original operative reports whenever possible. For most patients with systemic LV morphology, either HBP or LBBAP can be pursued depending on operator preference, but with the understanding that pacing electrical parameters are usually superior to the latter (see subsequent text). For patients with systemic RV morphology, HBP or very proximal LBBAP is usually attempted given the need for rapid engagement of the conduction system and maximally synchronous activation of the systemic RV.

Congenital Heart Disease with Systemic Left Ventricular Morphology

The overall implant approach (HBP versus LBBAP) for patients with systemic LV morphology should be contemplated in advance given the known limitations and advantages of each (**Table 1**). For HBP, a quadripolar catheter can be placed from the femoral vein before obtaining subclavian vein access to mark the precise position of the His bundle. Alternatively, this structure can be discovered by mapping with the pacing lead. Generally, delivery systems that provide sufficient access to the AV groove, as well as a secondary septal curvature are desirable for HBP. When His bundle potentials are observed on the unipolar sensing channel, the lead is rapidly rotated 3 to 4 turns to fixate the helix into the underlying ventricular myocardium. Acute pacing thresholds of less than 2 V at 1.0 ms are generally considered acceptable. Potential pitfalls of HSP include small R waves relative to the nearby atrial myocardium, a high ventricular pacing threshold, and lead

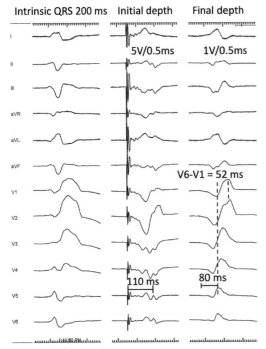

Intrinsic QRS 200 ms   Initial depth   Final depth

5V/0.5ms   1V/0.5ms

V6–V1 = 52 ms

110 ms   80 ms

Fig. 4. Representative example of left bundle branch pacing. Implant characteristics for the patient with tetralogy of Fallot and severe right ventricular enlargement from **Fig. 1** are shown. The baseline QRS morphology is complete right bundle branch block (RBBB) measuring 200 ms. With initial lead placement in the ventricular septum, an incomplete RBBB pattern is observed with a left ventricular activation time (LVAT) of 110 ms. With progressive advancement of the lead to the left ventricular endocardium, complete RBBB and abrupt shortening of the LVAT to 80 ms with V6–V1 interval of 52 ms develops, consistent with left bundle branch capture. The final QRS duration measures 170 ms.

instability. Given the relatively high risk of unacceptable sensing and pacing electrical parameters during follow up and lead dislodgement at this location, placement of a secondary ventricular lead when such patients are pacemaker dependent has been advocated.[14,15]

For LBBAP, a similar approach is used but additional steps are required to achieve proper lead positioning. Before lead placement, contrast delivery to visualize the overall boundaries of the morphologic RV is useful in CHD where distorted ventricular anatomy is common. Often, a coronary sinus lead delivery catheter is selectively cut to accommodate a second catheter with a secondary septal curve to provide optimal distal support and access to the septal RV. The delivery system is placed within the RV and rotated counterclockwise to position the catheter tip against the ventricular septum. With rapid clockwise rotation,

the lead is then driven into the ventricular septum in a left anterior oblique view or when necessary, more extreme angulation that best profiles the ventricular septum. Unipolar pacing to assess paced QRS morphology and pacing impedance as well as frequent contrast injections through the delivery catheter to gauge the distance that the lead has been advanced, are frequently used during lead fixation. When these measures suggest an LV septal location, no further rotation is undertaken to avoid perforation into the LV cavity (**Fig. 5**).

Congenital Heart Disease with Systemic Right Ventricular Morphology

For patients with CCTGA, both fluoroscopic-based and 3D mapping-guided approaches have been advocated and generally depend on operator preference and availability. Key advantages of 3D mapping include greater precision in lead placement and potential superiority in cases where the conduction tissues are arranged in an atypical manner.[16,17] The technique associated with HBP in this patient group is analogous to that described above, but often with a slightly less basal location of the His bundle and proximal left bundle branches. Although reasonable outcomes can be achieved with more distal CSP, rapid activation of the morphologic RV is best achieved when

Table 1
Relative advantages of His bundle versus left bundle area pacing in patients with congenital heart disease and systemic left ventricular morphology

His Bundle Pacing	Left Bundle Branch Area Pacing
Advantages	
• Greater anatomic familiarity	• High rate of successful implant
• Straightforward implant	• Lead stability
• Unequivocal capture assessment	• Excellent pacing electrical parameters
Disadvantages	
• Potential for lead instability	• Potential complications (perforation, coronary injury)
• Higher pacing threshold	• Steeper learning curve
• Potential atrial oversensing	• Lead extraction not described

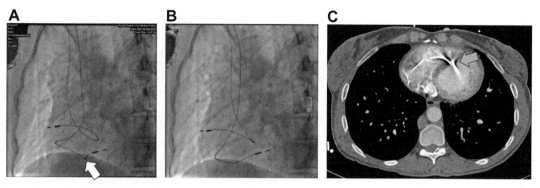

Fig. 5. Example of the fulcrum sign during left bundle branch pacing implantation. In this patient with left atrial isomerism and bilateral superior vena cava, a select secure lead has been placed over 10 mm into the interventricular septum, as verified by contrast injection. (*A*) and (*B*) Ventricular systole and diastole, respectively, the fulcrum sign is visible proximal to the lead insertion site of the lead into the ventricular septum (*white arrow*). (*C*) Location of the pacing lead by multi-slice computed tomography during routine follow up. The gray arrow denotes the location of the lead tip at the left ventricular endocardium.

pacing in the most basal position possible near the non-branching His bundle.[17]

DISCUSSION
Congenital Heart Disease with Systemic Left Ventricular Morphology

Among patients with CHD, CSP has been performed most frequently for the subgroup with systemic LV morphology. Initial studies demonstrated both feasibility and safety of this approach with no major complications and confirmed the durability of pacing electrical parameters over short follow-up periods.[18,19] More recently, these outcomes have been studied in the context of a systematic multicenter investigation.[20] Like the population with structurally normal

hearts, HBP as compared with LBBAP is associated with relatively higher ventricular pacing thresholds and diminished sensing at 1 year follow up. Such a finding is unsurprising, as the targeted conduction tissue for HBP is often located in close relationship to prior operative septal defect repair for many forms of CHD and may be partially encased in subendocardial fibrosis (**Fig. 6**). Most importantly, CSP seems to be at least equivalent to conventional CRT among CHD, with non-inferior improvement in LV systolic function and greater QRS shortening at 1 year after implant.[20] As such, CSP may be considered as an alternative to conventional CRT for CHD in situations where chronic ventricular pacing is anticipated or when RV pacing-induced cardiomyopathy has already developed.

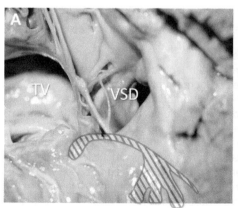
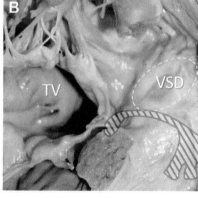

Fig. 6. Surgical scarring in relation to repaired ventricular septal defect and proximal conduction system in tetralogy of Fallot. (*A*) Unoperated ventricular septal defect (VSD) in a patient with tetralogy of Fallot. (*B*) Significant postoperative scarring is observed in the vicinity of the surgical patch. The putative course of the His bundle (hatched lines) is shown in a posteroinferior relationship relative to the VSD and may be encased in fibrosis, affecting long-term His bundle pacing outcomes.

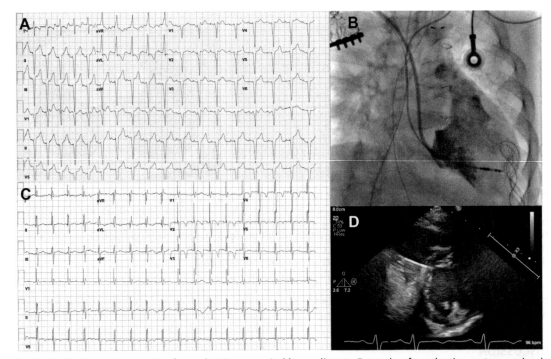

Fig. 7. Conduction system pacing for pediatric congenital heart disease. Example of conduction system pacing in a 9 year old girl with atrioventricular septal defect. (*A*) At baseline, the patient had a QRS duration of 140 ms with mild pacing-induced cardiomyopathy. (*B*) A right-sided implant approach was performed given prior left-sided device infection requiring extraction. Contrast injection outlines the limits of the right ventricular anatomy. (*C* and *D*) A Select Secure lead is placed deep into the ventricular septum where paced morphology was a QR pattern in V1 with a QRS duration of 90 ms and normalization of left ventricular ejection fraction.

Similar outcomes have also been noted for pediatric patients with CHD (**Fig. 7**).[18]

Congenital Heart Disease with Systemic Right Ventricular Morphology

CSP for patients with systemic RV morphology was first described in an adult patient with CCTGA.[21] Since then, numerous case reports as well as a larger, multicenter collaborative series[17] have described the outcomes of CSP for patients with CCTGA. Key findings from larger series are that electrical synchrony (as measured by the QRS duration) shortens significantly in those patients with baseline LV pacing and is preserved when CSP is pursued prophylactically. Additionally, pacing electrical parameters seem to remain excellent over time. Although sample sizes have been small and long-term outcomes are not yet available, acute symptomatic improvement in many patients undergoing HBP has been described.[17]

To date, experience with HBP among patients with DTGA and prior Mustard or Senning operation has been limited to isolated case reports. Although lead fixation at the proximal His bundle is desirable

for this anatomy, the procedure is particularly challenging because of the series of opposing curvatures through the innominate vein and superior venous baffle, and acute lead dislodgements have been reported. A right-sided implant strategy has been suggested by some to provide a more favorable approach to the ventricular septum in this anatomy.[19]

SUMMARY

Although the relative merits of CSP for CHD are increasingly understood, knowledge gaps remain. In particular, the optimal age at which to begin implantation of pediatric CSP is unknown, especially considering potential adverse effects on tricuspid valve function and collateral damage with penetration into the ventricular septum. Further, the outcomes of lead extraction involving deep septal myocardial leads are largely unknown and require further study.[22,23] Finally, the risks and benefits of HBP versus LBBAP and appropriate selection among CHD require further investigation. These and other issues will be best understood in the context of clinical trials or large registry databases with prospective data collection.

CLINICS CARE POINTS

- For systemic LV biventricular heart disease, CSP targets either the His bundle or LBB area and can provide similar benefit as compared with conventional CRT.
- Based on preliminary experience, LBBP seems to be associated with improved pacing electrical parameters as compared with HBP.
- For systemic RV biventricular heart disease, most clinical data support CSP for CCTGA with limited data available for DTGA after the Mustard or Senning operation.
- The distal His bundle or proximal LBB are reasonable targets for CCTGA.
- Limited data are also available for the use of CSP among pediatric patients with CHD; however, preliminary evidence suggests that this approach is reasonable and may be associated with a favorable risk/benefit profile as compared with conventional RV pacing.

REFERENCES

1. Salden F, Luermans J, Westra SW, et al. Short-term hemodynamic and electrophysiological effects of cardiac resynchronization by left ventricular septal pacing. J Am Coll Cardiol 2020;75:347–59.
2. Howard TS, Niu MC, Morris SA, et al. Right ventricular pacing after ventricular septal defect closure is associated with development of cardiac dysfunction. JACC Clin Electrophysiol 2020;6:348–50.
3. Huang W, Su L, Wu S, et al. A novel pacing strategy with low and stable output: pacing the left bundle branch immediately beyond the conduction block. Can J Cardiol 2017;33:1736 e1–e1736 e3.
4. Karpawich PP, Mital S. Comparative left ventricular function following atrial, septal, and apical single chamber heart pacing in the young. Pacing Clin Electrophysiol 1997;20:1983–8.
5. Kaye GC, Linker NJ, Marwick TH, et al. Effect of right ventricular pacing lead site on left ventricular function in patients with high-grade atrioventricular block: results of the Protect-Pace study. Eur Heart J 2015;36:856–62.
6. Hofferberth SC, Alexander ME, Mah DY, et al. Impact of pacing on systemic ventricular function in L-transposition of the great arteries. J Thorac Cardiovasc Surg 2016;151:131–8.
7. Yeo WT, Jarman JW, Li W, et al. Adverse impact of chronic subpulmonary left ventricular pacing on systemic right ventricular function in patients with congenitally corrected transposition of the great arteries. Int J Cardiol 2014;171:184–91.
8. Moore JP, Gallotti RG, Shannon KM, et al. A minimally invasive hybrid approach for cardiac resynchronization of the systemic right ventricle. Pacing Clin Electrophysiol 2019;42:171–7.
9. Davies MJ, Anderson RH, Becker AE. The Conduction System of the Heart. London, UK: Butterworths; 1983.
10. Vijayaraman P, Dandamudi G, Zanon F, et al. Permanent his bundle pacing: recommendations from a multicenter his bundle pacing collaborative working group for standardization of definitions, implant measurements, and follow-up. Heart Rhythm 2018; 15:460–8.
11. Wu S, Chen X, Wang S, et al. Evaluation of the criteria to distinguish left bundle branch pacing from left ventricular septal pacing. JACC Clin Electrophysiol 2021;7:1166–77.
12. Jastrzebski M, Burri H, Kielbasa G, et al. The V6-V1 interpeak interval: a novel criterion for the diagnosis of left bundle branch capture. Europace 2022;24:40–7.
13. Jastrzebski M, Kielbasa G, Curila K, et al. Physiology-based electrocardiographic criteria for left bundle branch capture. Heart Rhythm 2021;18:935–43.
14. Vijayaraman P, Naperkowski A, Subzposh FA, et al. Permanent His-bundle pacing: long-term lead performance and clinical outcomes. Heart Rhythm 2018;15:696–702.
15. Sharma PS, Dandamudi G, Herweg B, et al. Permanent His-bundle pacing as an alternative to biventricular pacing for cardiac resynchronization therapy: a multicenter experience. Heart Rhythm 2018;15:413–20.
16. Vijayaraman P, Mascarenhas V. Three-dimensional mapping-guided permanent His bundle pacing in a patient with corrected transposition of great arteries. HeartRhythm Case Rep 2019;5:600–2.
17. Moore JP, Gallotti R, Shannon KM, et al. Permanent conduction system pacing for congenitally corrected transposition of the great arteries: A Pediatric and Congenital Electrophysiology Society (PACES)/International Society for Adult Congenital Heart Disease (ISACHD) Collaborative Study. Heart Rhythm 2020;17:991–7.
18. Jimenez E, Zaban N, Sharma N, et al. His bundle and left bundle pacing in pediatrics and congenital heart disease: a single center experience. Pediatr Cardiol 2020;41:1425–31.
19. Cano Ó, Dandamudi G, Schaller RD, et al. Safety and feasibility of conduction system pacing in patients with congenital heart disease. J Cardiovasc Electrophysiol 2021;32:2692–703.
20. Moore JP, de Groot NMS, O'Connor M, et al. Conduction System Pacing Versus Conventional Cardiac Resynchronization Therapy in Congenital

Heart Disease. JACC Clin Electrophysiol 2023;9: 385–93.

21. Kean AC, Kay WA, Patel JK, et al. Permanent nonselective his bundle pacing in an adult with L-transposition of the great arteries and complete AV block. Pacing Clin Electrophysiol 2017;40:1313–7.

22. Vijayaraman P. Extraction of left bundle branch pacing lead. JACC Clin Electrophysiol 2020;6:903–4.

23. Ponnusamy SS, Vijayaraman P. Late dislodgement of left bundle branch pacing lead and successful extraction. J Cardiovasc Electrophysiol 2021;32: 2346–9.

Epicardial Devices in Pediatrics and Congenital Heart Disease

Reina Bianca Tan, MD[a],*, Elizabeth A. Stephenson, MD[b], Anica Bulic, MD[b]

KEYWORDS

- Pacemaker • Implantable cardioverter defibrillator • Cardiac implantable electronic device
- Epicardial

KEY POINTS

- Epicardial cardiac implantable electronic device (CIED) implant is more common in pediatrics due to size, body habitus, cardiovascular anatomy, and surgical repair.
- Lead dysfunction is more common in epicardial CIED systems as compared with transvenous devices.
- Defibrillation threshold testing still plays a role in pediatric and congenital heart disease patients as variation in patient size, anatomy, device configurations, and cardiac remodeling can lead to unpredictable vectors of defibrillation.

INTRODUCTION

Cardiac implantable electronic devices (CIEDs), including pacemakers (PM) and implantable cardiac defibrillators (ICDs), are indicated for a growing number of cardiac conditions.[1] Use of CIEDs in children and patients with congenital heart disease (CHD) has increased with ICD utilization more than doubling in recent years.[2] Specific challenges exist in CIED implantation in this population. Although there is an abundance of devices available, none are specifically designed for children and patients with CHD. Currently, there are no specific guidelines on best practice in device implantation given the scarcity of prospective studies.

Epicardial CIED systems possess advantages for children and patients with complex CHD as they do not rely on venous access, can be placed during concurrent surgery, and avoid endovascular leads. Endovascular leads carry with them associated thromboembolic risks, vascular risks, and infectious risks. However, these factors should be weighed against increased lead failure rates and pacing thresholds, as well as the more invasive surgery required for the placement of epicardial leads.

Pacemakers

Children with CHD are at risk for sinus node dysfunction and varying degrees of atrioventricular (AV) nodal block. This can be due to the nature of their structural heart disease, as in congenitally corrected transposition of the great arteries associated AV block, or surgically acquired. Despite advances in surgical techniques and perioperative care, the incidence of AV block in cardiopulmonary bypass surgeries remains approximately 2% to 3% in this current era, with 1% ultimately requiring a permanent PM system.[3] Permanent pacing is indicated in nonrecoverable surgical complete AV block as previous natural history studies have shown an increase in late mortality.[4] This leads to a not insignificant population of children with CHD with a CIED that complicates their care, can

[a] Division of Cardiology, Department of Pediatrics, NYU Langone Health and Hassenfeld Children's Hospital, 403 East 34th Street, Level 4, New York, NY 10017, USA; [b] University of Toronto, The Hospital for Sick Children, Labatt Family Heart Centre, 555 University Avenue, Room 1725, Toronto, Ontario M5G1X8, Canada
* Corresponding author. 403 East 34th Street, Level 4, New York, NY 10017.
E-mail address: reina.tan@nyulangone.org

Card Electrophysiol Clin 15 (2023) 467–480
https://doi.org/10.1016/j.ccep.2023.07.006
1877-9182/23/© 2023 Elsevier Inc. All rights reserved.

limit their activity and quality of life, and increases the number of hospital visits and procedures. Another population of patients are those with isolated congenital complete heart block. The unique features of being smaller and/or having structural heart disease necessitate much thought around how pediatric cardiologists and electrophysiologists decide on who receives a permanent pacing system, where the leads are placed, and how closely the patients are followed, appreciating the increased risk of complications in this vulnerable patient population.

Indications for permanent pacing were previously drawn from adult guidelines that were extrapolated and applied to the pediatric population. This was addressed recently by the publication of pediatric-focused guidelines on the implantation and management of CIEDs in the pediatric population.[5] With regard to postsurgical AV block, class I indications remain that a permanent PM is indicated in postoperative advanced second-degree or third-degree AV block that fails to recover by 7 to 10 days, or that does recover but has a late recurrence. Outside the context of surgery, certain forms of CHD have inherited risks of developing sinus node dysfunction or progressive AV block such that if bradycardia less than 60 to 70 bpm is noted along with consequential hemodynamic instability, an appropriate permanent PM is indicated. In isolated congenital complete heart block, class I indication in asymptomatic neonates and infants now focus on mean ventricular rate of less than 50 bpm. See **Table 1** for a comprehensive list of CIED implantation recommendations.

Epicardial pacemaker system and implantation
Epicardial pacing systems are more often used in the pediatric and CHD population compared with the adults. There are various reasons for this, which include small caliber of venous anatomy with high risk of venous occlusion; venous anatomy that precludes a transvenous approach due to either anomalous drainage, stenosis or occlusion; or intracardiac shunts or single ventricle physiology that confers an inappropriately high risk of thromboembolic events. There is no clear cut-off as to what the smallest patient age, weight, and height are safe for transvenous PM implantation. Technically, there have been reports of transvenous systems implanted in children 10 kg or less, but with significant device revisions needed in the acute to intermediate periods.[6,7] The decision as to which type of pacing system to place in children less than 20 kg should be made on a case-by-case basis and is institutionally dependent. The presence of intracardiac shunts or single ventricle physiology is generally a contraindication

for transvenous PM implantation due to a 2-fold greater risk of systemic thromboembolism.[8]

The epicardial pacing system consists of a pulse generator or "can," which houses a battery and circuitry, attached to lead(s). The most common epicardial lead used is a steroid-eluting bipolar lead (Model 4968 CapSure Epi, Medtronic Inc., Minneapolis, MN, USA), which has shown good long-term outcomes in terms of lead survival and acceptable lead parameters.[9,10] Leads can vary in terms of pacing configuration (eg, unipolar vs bipolar), method by which the leads are affixed to the myocardium (eg, screw-in vs sutured-on), and whether they are steroid eluting versus nonsteroid eluting. Steroid-eluting epicardial leads have been shown to have lower implant and chronic thresholds compared with nonsteroid eluting leads, and comparable but slightly higher than transvenous leads.[11] The surgical approach to implanting epicardial PM leads is either via median sternotomy, subxiphoid, or lateral thoracotomy.

The location of the epicardial ventricular lead is arguably the most important implant consideration. It is well established in the literature that ventricular pacing has several deleterious cellular and histologic effects. It can cause distortion of myofiber size and morphology, fibrosis, sclerosis, fatty infiltration, and mitochondrial morphologic changes.[12] A suboptimal ventricular lead location can lead to electromechanical dyssynchrony and consequentially a higher risk of pacing-induced cardiomyopathy. This is an even greater risk in CHD where residual pressure and/or volume-loading lesions make the myocardium even more vulnerable to dysfunction. Left ventricle (LV) apical and mid-lateral wall pacing has borne out to be the optimal site for permanent ventricular pacing in terms of preserving LV synchrony and systolic function.[13-15] The least desirable location is the right ventricle (RV) apex and anterior free wall, which has consistently shown long-term risk of LV remodeling, dyssynchrony, and dysfunction.

Pacemaker complications
Epicardial steroid-eluting leads have a reasonable longevity, with 1-, 2-, and 5-year lead survival at 96%, 90%, and 74%, respectively.[16] Lead failure rates are reported as high as 16%, with the most common cause being increased thresholds, followed by lead fracture and rarely phrenic or muscle stimulation or inappropriate sensing. They have comparable sensing to transvenous leads but higher pacing thresholds at all time points, potentially draining the battery and hastening generator exchanges and increasing the number of procedures.[11]

Coronary artery compression and cardiac strangulation are rare yet life-threatening complications

Table 1
Indications for permanent pacemaker implantation in pediatrics

Recommendations	Class	LOE
Postoperative Atrioventricular Block		
Permanent pacemaker implantation is indicated for postoperative advanced second- or third-degree AV block that persists for at least 7–10 d after cardiac surgery.	I	B-NR
Permanent pacemaker implantation is indicated for late-onset advanced second- or third-degree AV block especially when there is a prior history of transient postoperative AV block.	I	C-LD
Permanent pacemaker implantation may be considered for unexplained syncope in patients with a history of transient postoperative advanced second- or third-degree AV block.	IIb	C-LD
Permanent pacemaker implantation may be considered at <7 postoperative days when advanced second- or third-degree AV block is not expected to resolve due to extensive injury to the cardiac conduction system.	IIb	C-EO
Permanent pacemaker implantation may be considered in select patients with transient postoperative advanced second- or third-degree AV block who are predisposed to progressive conduction abnormalities.	IIb	C-EO
Congenital Heart Disease		
Permanent pacemaker implantation is indicated for CCAVB in neonates or infants with complex CHD when bradycardia is associated with hemodynamic compromise or when the mean ventricular rate is <60–70 bpm.	I	C-LD
Permanent pacemaker implantation with atrial anti-tachycardia pacing is reasonable for patients with CHD and recurrent episodes of intra-atrial re-entrant tachycardia when catheter ablation and medication are ineffective or not acceptable treatments.	IIa	B-NR
Permanent atrial or dual-chamber pacemaker implantation is reasonable for patients with CHD and impaired hemodynamics due to sinus bradycardia or loss of AV synchrony.	IIa	C-LD
Permanent atrial or dual-chamber pacing is reasonable for patients with tachy–brady syndrome and symptoms attributable to pauses due to sudden-onset bradycardia.	IIa	C-LD
Permanent pacemaker implantation is reasonable for sinus or junctional bradycardia with *complex* CHD when the mean awake resting heart rate is <40 bpm or when there are prolonged pauses in the ventricular rate.	IIa	C-EO
Permanent pacing may be considered for sinus or junctional bradycardia with *simple or moderate* CHD when the mean awake resting heart rate is <40 bpm or when there are prolonged pauses in the ventricular rate.	IIb	C-EO
Endocardial leads should be avoided in patients with CHD and intracardiac shunt except in select cases, for whom there should be an individualized consideration of the risk/benefit ratio. In these exceptional cases anticoagulation is mandatory, but thromboembolism remains a risk.	III Harm	B-NR
Isolated Congenital Complete Atrioventricular Block		
Permanent pacemaker implantation is indicated for patients with congenital complete atrioventricular block (CCAVB) with symptomatic bradycardia.	I	B-NR

(continued on next page)

Table 1
(continued)

Recommendations	Class	LOE
Permanent pacemaker implantation is indicated for patients with CCAVB with a wide QRS escape rhythm, complex ventricular ectopy, or ventricular dysfunction.	I	B-NR
Permanent pacemaker implantation is indicated for CCAVB in asymptomatic neonates or infants when the mean ventricular rate is ≤50 bpm. Ventricular rate alone should not be used as implant criteria, as symptoms due to low cardiac output may occur at faster heart rates.	I	C-LD
Permanent pacemaker implantation is reasonable for asymptomatic CCAVB beyond the first year of life when the mean ventricular rate is <50 bpm or there are prolonged pauses in ventricular rate.	IIa	B-NR
Permanent pacemaker implantation is reasonable for CCAVB with left ventricular dilation (z score ≥3) associated with significant mitral insufficiency or systolic dysfunction.	IIa	C-LD
Permanent pacemaker implantation may be considered for CCAVB in asymptomatic adolescents with an acceptable ventricular rate, a narrow QRS complex, and normal ventricular function, based on an individualized consideration of the risk/benefit ratio.	IIb	C-LD

From Maully J. Shah et al., 2021 PACES Expert Consensus Statement on the Indications and Management of Cardiovascular Implantable Electronic Devices in Pediatric Patients, Heart Rhythm, 18 (11), 2021, 1888-1924, https://doi.org/10.1016/j.hrthm.2021.07.038.

of epicardial pacing and defibrillation leads. The true incidence and prevalence are unknown and likely underestimated due to the lack of a high index of clinical suspicion and systematic screening. Previously, only case reports were reported in the literature with variable clinical presentation including incidental murmur, fatigue, chest pain, syncope, and sudden death.[17] In the largest series thus far, coronary artery compression was found in 5.5% of pediatric and adult patients with epicardial leads who were undergoing coronary angiography or computerized tomography (CT) for various reasons.[18] Although most of them were symptomatic, 25% were asymptomatic, highlighting the necessity for surveillance. It is good practice to obtain a 2-view chest X-ray post-operatively to document baseline epicardial lead position to ensure there is no excessive lead encircling the heart. Although the patient is growing, it might be prudent to obtain surveillance chest X-rays every 1 to 2 years to screen for leads encircling the heart or large lead loops coursing over a coronary artery territory. Even if the chest X-ray is reassuring, if a patient presents with concerning symptoms as listed above or unexplained ventricular dysfunction, there should be little hesitation in moving forward with either a cardiac CT or coronary angiography to screen for coronary artery perfusion defects since the sensitivity of chest X-rays is low.

Patients with CHD often require cardiac MRI scans for volumetric and flow data, or other solid organ scans. The existence of an epicardial CIED system is currently a contraindication for MRI scans, whether the system is intact or abandoned leads. Recent data have suggested that in fact, MRI scans in select patients with no other diagnostic imaging modality present can be performed safely.[19,20] Rare complications included mild discomfort at the CIED site without any clinically significant permanent changes to the PM incurred.

Implantable cardiac defibrillator
Implantable cardioverter defibrillators (ICDs) have long been recognized in their role for primary and secondary prevention of sudden death secondary to ventricular tachycardia (VT) or ventricular fibrillation (VF).[21,22] There is an increased risk of ventricular arrhythmias in patients with repaired congenital cardiac disease, primary electrical disease such as the long QT syndrome, catecholaminergic ventricular tachycardia, Brugada syndrome, and idiopathic ventricular fibrillation, as well as hypertrophic and dilated cardiomyopathies. ICD implantation, applied with careful risk assessment, has been shown to improve outcomes and decrease mortality in pediatric patients and in patients with CHD who are found to be at high risk for ventricular arrhythmias.[2,21–24] In patients with CHD, appropriate ICD shock rates of 3% to 6% per year have been shown, with an even higher frequency of appropriate shocks when the device is placed for secondary prevention. However, the optimal ICD system implantation technique in small children and patients with

Table 2
Indications for implantable cardioverter defibrillator implantation in pediatrics

Recommendations	Class	LOE
ICD implantation is indicated for survivors of SCA due to VT/VF if completely reversible causes have been excluded and an ICD is considered to be more beneficial than alternative treatments that may significantly reduce the risk of SCA.	I	B-NR
ICD implantation may be considered for patients with sustained VT that cannot be adequately controlled with medication and/or catheter ablation.	IIb	C-EO
ICD therapy may be considered for primary prevention of SCD in patients with genetic cardiovascular diseases and risk factors for SCA or pathogenic mutations and family history of recurrent SCA.	IIb	C-EO
Long QT Syndrome (LQTS)		
ICD implantation along with the use of beta-blockade is indicated for patients with a diagnosis of LQTS who are survivors of SCA. In select LQTS patients, medical therapy and/or cardiac sympathetic denervation may be considered as an alternative.	I	B-NR
ICD implantation is indicated in LQTS patients with symptoms (arrhythmic syncope or VT) in whom beta-blockade is either ineffective or not tolerated and cardiac sympathetic denervation or other medications are not considered effective alternatives.	I	B-NR
ICD therapy may be considered for primary prevention in LQTS patients with established clinical risk factors and/or pathogenic mutations.	II	C-LD
Catecholaminergic Polymorphic Ventricular Tachycardia (CPVT)		
ICD implantation is indicated in patients with a diagnosis of CPVT who experience cardiac arrest or arrhythmic syncope despite maximally tolerated beta-blocker plus flecainide and/or cardiac sympathetic denervation.	I	C-LD
ICD implantation is reasonable in combination with pharmacologic therapy with or without cardiac sympathetic denervation when aborted SCA is the initial presentation of CPVT. Pharmacologic therapy and/or cardiac sympathetic denervation without ICD may be considered as an alternative.	IIa	C-LD
ICD implantation may be considered in CPVT patients with polymorphic/bidirectional VT despite optimal pharmacologic therapy with or without cardiac sympathetic denervation.	IIb	C-LD
Brugada Syndrome (BrS)		
ICD implantation is indicated in patients with a diagnosis of BrS who are survivors of SCA or have documented spontaneous sustained VT.	I	B-NR
ICD implantation is reasonable for patients with BrS with a spontaneous type I Brugada ECG pattern and recent syncope presumed due to ventricular arrhythmias.	IIa	B-NR
ICD implantation may be considered in patients with syncope presumed due to ventricular arrhythmias with a type I Brugada ECG pattern only with provocative medications.	IIb	C-EO
Hypertrophic Cardiomyopathy (HCM)		
ICD implantation is indicated in patients with HCM who are survivors of SCA or have spontaneous sustained VT.	I	B-NR
For children with HCM who have 1 primary risk factors, including unexplained syncope, massive left ventricular hypertrophy, nonsustained VT, or family history of early HCM-related SCD, ICD placement is reasonable after considering the potential complications of long-term ICD placement.	IIa	B-NR

(continued on next page)

Table 2
(continued)

Recommendations	Class	LOE
ICD implantation may be considered in patients with HCM without the above risk factors but with secondary risk factors for SCA such extensive late gadolinium enhancement (LGE) on cardiac MRI or systolic dysfunction.	IIb	B-NR
Arrhythmogenic Cardiomyopathy (ACM)		
ICD implantation is indicated in patients with ACM who have been resuscitated from SCA or sustained VT that is not hemodynamically tolerated.	I	B-NR
ICD implantation is reasonable in patients with ACM with hemodynamically tolerated sustained VT, syncope presumed due to ventricular arrhythmia, or an left ventricular ejection fraction (LVEF) 35%.	IIa	B-NR
ICD implantation may be considered in patients with inherited ACM associated with increased risk of SCD based on an assessment of additional risk factors.	IIb	C-LD
Nonischemic Dilated Cardiomyopathy		
ICD implantation is indicated in patients with non ischemic dilated cardiomyopathy (NIDCM) who either survive SCA or experience sustained VT not due to completely reversible causes.	I	B-NR
ICD implantation may be considered in patients with NIDCM and syncope or an LVEF 35%, despite optimal medical therapy.	IIb	C-LD
Congenital Heart Disease		
ICD implantation is indicated for CHD patients who are survivors of SCA after evaluation to define the cause of the event and exclude any completely reversible causes.	I	B-NR
ICD implantation is indicated for CHD patients with hemodynamically unstable sustained VT who have undergone hemodynamic and electrophysiologic evaluation. Catheter ablation or surgical repair may be possible alternatives in carefully selected patients.	I	C-LD
ICD implantation is reasonable for CHD patients with systemic LVEF 35% and sustained VT or presumed arrhythmogenic syncope.	IIa	C-LD
ICD implantation may be considered for CHD patients with spontaneous hemodynamically stable sustained VT who have undergone hemodynamic and electrophysiologic evaluation. Catheter ablation or surgical repair may be possible alternatives in carefully selected patients.	IIb	C-EO
ICD implantation may be considered for CHD patients with unexplained syncope in the presence of ventricular dysfunction, nonsustained VT, or inducible ventricular arrhythmias at electrophysiologic study.	IIb	C-LD
ICD implantation may be considered for CHD patients with a single or systemic right ventricular ejection fraction <35%, particularly in the presence of additional risk factors such as VT, arrhythmic syncope, or severe systemic AV valve insufficiency.	IIb	C-EO

From Maully J. Shah et al., 2021 PACES Expert Consensus Statement on the Indications and Management of Cardiovascular Implantable Electronic Devices in Pediatric Patients, Heart Rhythm, 18 (11), 2021, 1888-1924, https://doi.org/10.1016/j.hrthm.2021.07.038.

CHD with limited venous access has not been well defined, despite advances in ICD technology and ICD leads.

Pediatric recommendations for ICD implantation have been primarily based on adult data and, with some modifications, applied to younger patients. The 2021 PACES Expert Consensus Statement on CIED management in pediatric patients is based on limited clinical data combined with expert opinion and consensus, and thus requires the application of case-specific clinical judgment and a shared decision-making approach.[5] The recommendations from that Consensus Statement are summarized in **Table 2**.

ICD implantations in children and patients with CHD frequently require nonstandard device and lead implantation techniques, as well as multiple procedures over a lifetime. The most obvious differences in need for defibrillator systems in children are related to size. The relatively large generator size and lead diameter and length make implantation challenging. As is seen with PM implantations, size constraints due to small vasculature in young children and abnormal venous and intracardiac anatomy in patients with CHD may preclude transvenous lead placement. The patient's cardiac anatomy, prior surgical and interventional procedures, existing supraventricular and ventricular tachyarrhythmias, and the requirement for future intervention all play a substantial role when deciding on the ideal ICD system. Other important considerations include shock strength, programming issues, and overlap of tachycardia detection criteria with normal pediatric heart rates.

The first-generation epicardial ICD system used patch/es sutured outside or inside the pericardium in the epicardium. The standard configuration when one patch was implanted was the patch sewn to the parietal pericardium in the region of the left ventricular apex. When 2 patches were used, the cathodal lead was sewn to pericardium over the posterolateral region of the left ventricle and the anodal lead was placed inferiorly over the diaphragmatic aspects of the ventricles.[25] The epicardial defibrillation patches originally consisted of a semirigid titanium mesh embedded in a plastic square (CPI, Cardiac Pacemaker Inc.). Later patch electrodes were made of a drawn brazed strand cable as conductor, titanium as patch mesh material, and silicone rubber for external insulation (model 67, Cardiac Pacemakers Inc., St. Paul, MN, USA) or a multifilar MP35N alloy conductor and platinum alloy mesh material with a silicone rubber insulation (model 6897/6921, Medtronic Inc.).

Pediatric patients were previously limited to epicardial systems due to the anthropometric issues, longitudinal growth, ICD size, large size of the transvenous electrode, and inappropriate shocking coil spacing.[26] Even with improvements in transvenous ICD electrodes, epicardial placement remains the preferred method for smaller children.

The decision to implant an epicardial system is provider and institution dependent. Most would opt for epicardial ICD system in patients less than 15 to 20 kg, but body habitus must also be considered. Other common reasons for epicardial implant include the presence of any intracardiac shunts due to risk of paradoxical emboli, presence of cardiac baffles limiting vascular access to the heart the presence of venous occlusion or stenosis, history of recurrent venous thrombosis, history of recurrent device infections or infective endocarditis, smaller subclavian vein, and superior vena cava size due to the presence of a persistent left superior vena cava.

In patients undergoing planned cardiac surgery and meeting criteria for ICD, an epicardial implant may be considered as there is minimal additional procedure time. However, a particular challenge with epicardial lead implantation is the presence of epicardial fat, adhesions, and fibrosis, particularly in patients with CHD who have had prior cardiac surgeries. Widespread epicardial fibrosis makes the procedure technically difficult and sometimes unfeasible due to unacceptable thresholds.

Implantable cardiac defibrillator system configurations and implantation

Various implant techniques have been described for children and adults with CHD.[27–30] The epicardial ICD system consists of a defibrillation patch or coil, pulse generator, and bipolar pace-sense lead/s. An epicardial PM lead is placed on the ventricle for sensing and pacing, and the pulse generator serves as an active can. Unipolar pacing leads are generally avoided due to the increased potential for oversensing, resulting in inappropriate ICD shocks. The shock coil is positioned to ensure that maximum ventricular myocardial mass is in the shock vector between the shock electrode and the pulse generator. The exact location of this will depend on the cardiac anatomy and must be individualized in patients with CHD.

Often novel off-label use and improvisation is necessary. Apart from the epicardial patch electrodes (**Fig. 1**A), subcutaneous arrays or transvenous ICD (**Fig. 1**A-C) coils can be used as the high voltage (HV) coil.[2,27,28] Subcutaneous array and coils were originally designed for adjunctive use to lower the defibrillation threshold. Transvenous ICD leads, superior vena cava leads, or subcutaneous coils have also been used for this purpose.

Surgical approach options for epicardial ICD implant include median sternotomy, left lateral (mini-) thoracotomy, and subxiphoid access. Schneider and colleagues[31] reported success using a minimally invasive technique via an inframammary thoracotomy with epicardial pace/sense lead implant and defibrillation coil placed posterior to the pericardial sac.

Early epicardial ICD systems used epicardial defibrillation patch/es sutured to the epicardium or pericardium (see **Fig. 1**A). Patches sutured to the pericardium resulted in less patch distortion.

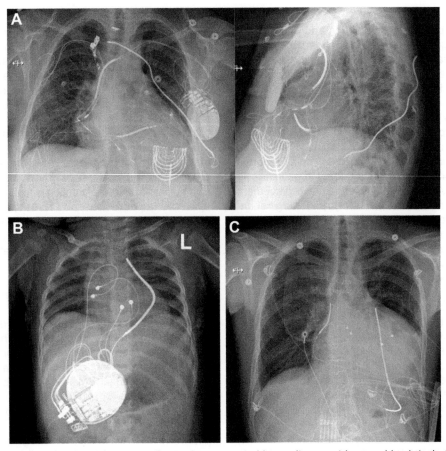

Fig. 1. High voltage leads. (*A*) Patient with complex congenital heart disease with several leads including abandoned leads in place consistent of an epicardial defibrillator patch, dual chamber transvenous ICD system with several abandoned transvenous leads, and a subcutaneous coil posteriorly. (*B*) Infant with a dual chamber ICD system. Bipolar epicardial leads for sensing and transvenous ICD coil implanted in epicardial position. (*C*) Patient with Ebstein anomaly post repair and bidirectional Glenn with a dual chamber ICD system. Bipolar epicardial leads for sensing, transvenous SVC coil placed along the right SVC and subcutaneous coil placed posteriorly.

This approach was associated with a high incidence of complications resulting in significant early and late morbidity and often unfavorable defibrillation threshold (DFTs), which is discussed further below.[23,32,33] Currently, nontraditional surgical methods of implantation have been described, using off-label use of standard transvenous single or dual coil HV leads, or the subcutaneous defibrillator lead 6996-SQ (Medtronic) or the subcutaneous 3-limb Endotak SQ array (Boston Scientific). In the structurally normal heart, the ICD coils are actively fixed to the pericardium either in the posterior mediastinal space medially, along the lateral left ventricular wall laterally, or posteriorly behind the ventricular mass (**Fig. 2**A). The coil can also be placed in the pleural space (**Fig. 2**B) or in an extra-pleural location between the thoracic wall and the parietal pleura (**Fig. 2**). As mentioned above, the ideal location of the HV lead is dependent on the cardiac anatomy and should

place the bulk of the ventricular myocardium between the coil and the generator to create the best vector for defibrillation. In our practice, the electrophysiologist is present during device implant to ensure appropriate lead placement and testing.

The generator is positioned in the abdominal wall within the rectus muscle sheath or in a prepectoral position. Others opt to place the device in a subcardial position, particularly in the smallest children where a submuscular device may remain at risk of erosion. The generator is placed horizontally either in a pocket between the diaphragm and the parietal pericardium or in the pericardial cavity in contact with the diaphragmatic surface of the heart and fixed to prevent migration of the device.

The novel or alternative configurations have been used successfully in children and young adults with CHD. However, these patients require close monitoring and follow-up, including routine testing of the defibrillation threshold, as they are

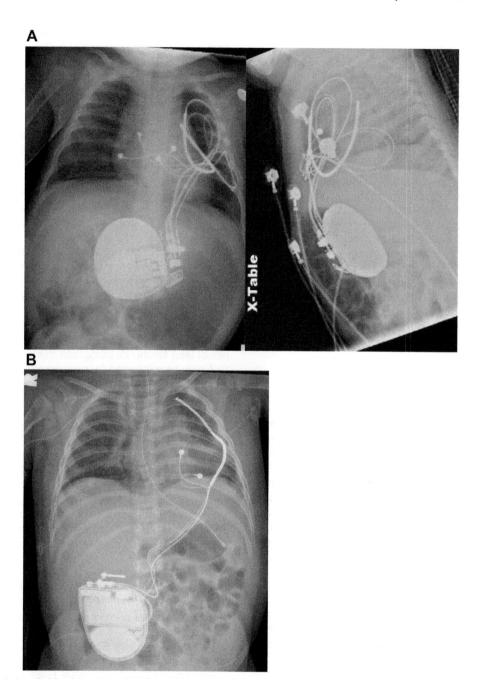

Fig. 2. Epicardial lead position. (*A*) ICD coil in pericardial position. (*B*) ICD coil in pleural space.

nonstandard technologies and are known to be prone to unanticipated complications, particularly hardware complications.

Implantable cardiac defibrillator testing

Successful defibrillation occurs when a large voltage gradient disrupts the eddy currents and allows uniform depolarization. Based on the critical mass hypothesis, the defibrillation threshold is reached when a sufficient mass of excitable cells

is simultaneously depolarized, thus interrupting activation wavefronts. DFT testing attempts to determine the likelihood of converting out of ventricular fibrillation. The threshold at which this gradient exists is recognized to be dynamic, and thus the test is probabilistic in nature. Defibrillation safety margin (DSM) is the lowest successful energy tested during defibrillation testing. An inadequate DSM is typically defined as a <10 J difference between the lowest successful energy tested during DSM testing and the maximum output of the ICD generator being used.[34,35]

DFTs used to be routinely performed at every ICD implant, prior to discharge and at follow-up intervals. Adult centers caring for patients with structurally normal hearts have been moving away from this practice as potential complications of DFT testing and shocks are increasingly recognized, and standard transvenous ICDs in adult patients have become more reliable with modern iterations. In pediatric and CHD patients, however, the variation in patient size, heterogeneous anatomy, generator-to-coil configurations, myocardial hypertrophy, and cardiac remodeling post-surgical or intervention procedure can potentially lead to unpredictable vectors of defibrillation in this group of patients.[22,36] In patients with a high DFT, the shock vector can be changed, or the addition of a subcutaneous high voltage lead or array can achieve an acceptable margin for defibrillation. DSM testing for patients with CHD has also seen a decline in recent years and appears to be safe.[35]

Implantable cardiac defibrillator-related complications

Epicardial and pericardial ICD leads have a shorter life expectancy than typical endocardial ICD systems.[37] Several studies have showed that within a follow-up period of 2 years, lead system revisions were required in ~25% of patients.[38–40] Lead failure in children typically results from physical activity, growth-related distortion, and unfavorable position in terms of exposure to physical impact. These have resulted in a substantial number of lead fractures or dislodgement of electrodes which can result in inappropriate shocks. A recent study of CIEDs in adults with CHD showed the incidence of CIED dysfunction was similar for transvenous and epicardial implants.[41]

Complications can be broken down into categories including procedural complications, therapy complications, lead-related complications, and others, as we explore below.

Implantable cardiac defibrillator implantation procedure-related complications Data on the incidence of epicardial system-specific procedural complications are limited. Various studies looking at complications in both transvenous and non-transvenous ICD systems show procedural complication rates between 15% and 26%.[22,37] These include pocket infection, hematoma, lead dislodgement, and post-pericardiotomy syndrome related to epicardial lead implantation. Tonko and colleagues[41] recently published a small series of 11 patients with epicardial ICD systems.

Perioperative complications unrelated to concomitant cardiac surgery occurred in 2 patients: one was due to epicardial lead displacement 7 days postprocedure requiring re-operation and the other to elevated DFT resulting in addition of a subcutaneous coil.

Inappropriate implantable cardiac defibrillator therapy Inappropriate ICD discharges create significant morbidity and are more common in pediatric patients compared with adults, occurring at a rate of up to 1.3 shocks per year of follow-up.[23] Expressed in percentages of ICD recipients, current adult ICD systems deliver inappropriate shocks in only 4% at 3 years of follow-up compared with 13% to 50% in the pediatric population.[2,5,21–24] Patients with CHD also have a higher rate of inappropriate shocks compared with the non-CHD population. Inappropriate shocks have been attributed to higher heart rates in children, supraventricular tachycardia (SVT), T-wave oversensing, as well as from the increased risk of lead failure. Inappropriate therapies due to SVT may be minimized by programming changes such as increasing the detection threshold and use of discrimination algorithms, as well as usage of β-blockers. In children old enough to participate, performing an exercise stress test to determine the maximum heart rate may be helpful to ensure that sinus tachycardia does not exceed the tachycardia detection threshold.[42] These maneuvers however cannot prevent inappropriate shocks due to lead failure. Frequent inappropriate shocks are a major issue as they can result in a painful experience and sometimes post-traumatic stress disorder in the affected children and adolescents.

Defibrillation lead-specific complications Lead complications occur in 15% to 30%.[23,24,43] Earlier lead failures are likely related to increased activity and lead stress, as well as the longer life span with the ICD in the young. Some studies have shown CHD to be a risk factor.[5,21,22]

Epicardial ICD patches have been associated with fracture and crinkling of patches, rise in DFT, and deterioration in system performance. A relatively high rate of epicardial patch fracture is seen patients with CHD.[44] There have been also reports of rare but severe occurrences of constrictive pericarditis.[45–47] Studies comparing lead survival in contemporary epicardial ICD versus endocardial systems in pediatrics and CHD are limited. A recent study comparing CIED systems (PM and ICD) in adult CHD patients showed the incidence of CIED system dysfunction and reinterventions are similar however lead dysfunction is more common in

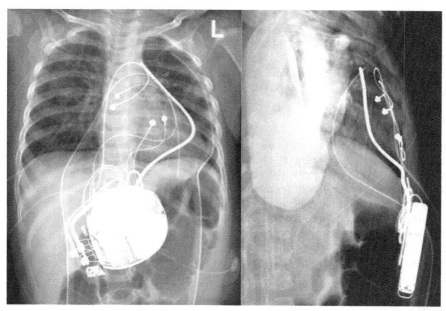

Fig. 3. ICD lead dislodgment. Post implant, ICD coil migrated into the pocket and came into contact with the generator necessitating revision of the system.

epicardial systems.[48] Adult studies in patients with structurally normal hearts have shown no significant differences in lead complication rates between endocardial and epicardial systems. However, epicardial systems were associated with higher perioperative mortality.[49]

Nontraditional epicardial systems using subcutaneous or transvenous as high voltage coil systems are subject to lead dislodgement, epicardial lead fracture, and insulation break. Rarely, the dislodgement of the ICD coil can lead to contact with the generator necessitating revision of the system, and thus caution with securing the lead and generator is important (**Fig. 3**). There is an increased rate of lead malfunction, particularly in young patients. Patients with a body surface area less than 1.2 m² had a 4.5-fold increased risk for lead failures.[50]

Implantable cardiac defibrillator generator-specific complications The most frequent indication for generator replacement is when the generator reaches elective replacement interval. However, manufacturer's safety advisories and device recall also may result in unanticipated interventions, hospitalizations, and morbidity.

Increase in defibrillation thresholds In pediatric patients, the failure rate of first ICD shock (both transvenous and nontransvenous) to terminate ventricular arrhythmia has been reported to be as high as 7% in one study as compared to a rate of 3.1% in adults.[51] This has been attributed to a chronic rise in defibrillation threshold, as well as shifting vectors due to growth. Although epicardial ICD systems are effective, these novel ICD systems tend to have higher defibrillation thresholds. Rise in defibrillation energy requirement over time has been noted in pediatric and adult congenital patients. Stephenson and colleagues[38] showed that during routine DFT testing in patients with epicardial or novel ICD configurations, 12% had clinically significant changes that required ICD reprogramming or hardware revision at a mean duration of 32 ± 23 months after ICD implantation. A more intensified device follow-up should be considered due to reported higher failure rate secondary to lead movement, elevated DFT, or early failure.

Psychosocial impact The psychosocial impact of ICD therapy has been well reported. In children with ICDs, some studies have shown signs of generalized depression and/or anxiety in 44%, whereas clinical depression was seen in 12% in another study.[52,53] A recent study looking at the incidence of post-traumatic stress disorder (PTSD) showed 12% of pediatric patients met the screening criteria for a likely PTSD diagnosis as compared to 47% for parents.[54] In adult patients with ICDs, PTSD rates can be as high as 14% to 36%.[55]

Health-related quality of life for children (HRQoL) with CIEDs is lower when compared with healthy controls. However, most have normal proxy- and self-reported disease-specific HRQoL. There is a trend toward higher risk for low disease-specific

HRQoL in younger patients, ICD patients, and patients with a structural CHD.[56]

Special attention should be given to these patients and caregivers. Timely evaluation can identify patients or parents who may benefit from psychological support.

SUMMARY

Epicardial cardiac rhythm devices in pediatrics and adults with CHD are effective and lifesaving. Complications include lead dysfunction, cardiac strangulation, and rising defibrillation thresholds. Inappropriate shocks remain a significant risk in ICDs. In patients with CHD, implant may be more complex and requires training and experience in CHD. These procedures are best performed in specialized pediatric and adult CHD centers. Device programming should be tailored for each patient to avoid inappropriate therapy or ICD shocks.

CLINICS CARE POINTS

- The location of the epicardial ventricular lead is important in preventing pacing-induced cardiomyopathy.
- LV apical and mid-lateral are the most optimal site for permanent ventricular pacing in terms of preserving LV synchrony and systolic function.
- Unipolar pacing leads are generally avoided in epicardial ICD systems due to the increased potential for oversensing, resulting in inappropriate ICD shocks.
- The shock coil location depends on the cardiac anatomy and must be individualized in patients with CHD as it is important to ensure that maximum ventricular myocardial mass is in the shock vector between the shock electrode and the pulse generator.
- DFT/DSM testing should be considered in pediatric and CHD patients as variation in patient size, heterogeneous anatomy, generator-to-coil configurations, myocardial hypertrophy, and cardiac remodeling post-surgical or intervention procedure can potentially lead to unpredictable vectors of defibrillation.

DISCLOSURE

None of the authors have any significant affiliations or relationships with commercial enterprise or any other potential conflicts of interest.

REFERENCES

1. Joy PS, Kumar G, Poole JE, et al. Cardiac implantable electronic device infections: who is at greatest risk? Heart Rhythm 2017;6:839–45.
2. Alexander ME, Cecchin F, Walsh EP, et al. Implications of implantable cardioverter defibrillator therapy in congenital heart disease and pediatrics. J Cardiovasc Electrophysiol 2004;15:72–6.
3. Romer AJ, Tabbutt S, Etheride SP, et al. Atrioventricular block after congenital heart surgery: analysis from the pediatric cardiac critical care Consortium. J Thorac Cardiovasc Surg 2019;157(3):1168–77.
4. Krongrad E. Prognosis for patients with congenital heart disease and postoperative intraventricular conduction defects. Circulation 1978;57:867–70.
5. Writing Committee Members, Shah MJ, Silka MJ, Silva JNA, et al. 2021 PACES expert consensus Statement on the indications and management of cardiovascular implantable electronic devices in pediatric patients. Heart Rhythm 2021 Nov;18(11):1888–924.
6. Kammeraad JAE, Rosenthal E, Bostock J, et al. Endocardia pacemaker implantation in infants weighing < or = 10 kilograms. Pacing Clin Electrophysiol 2004;11:1466–74.
7. Konta L, Chubb MH, Bostock J, et al. Twenty-seven years experience with transvenous pacemaker implantation in children weighing <10 kg. Circ Arrhythm Electrophysiol 2016;9:e003422.
8. Khairy P, Landzberg MJ, Gatzoulis MA, et al. Transvenous pacing leads and systemic thromboemboli in patients with intracardiac shunts: a multicenter study. Circulation 2006;113:2391–7.
9. Paech C, Kostelka M, Dahnert I, et al. Performance of steroid eluting bipolar epicardial leads in pediatric and congenital haert disease patients: 15 years of single center experience. J Cardiothorac Surg 2014;9:84–9.
10. Beaufort-Krol GC, Mulder H, Nagelkerke D, et al. Comparison of longevity, pacing, and sensing characteristics of steroid-eluting epicardial versus conventional endocardial pacing leads in children. J Thorac Cardiovasc Surg 1999;3:523–8.
11. Fortescue EB, Berul CI, Cecchin F, et al. Comparison of modern steroid-eluting epicardial and thin transvenous pacemaker leads in pediatric and congenital heart disease patients. J Interv Card Electrophysiol 2005;14(1):27–36.
12. Karpawich PP, Rabah R, Haas JE. Altered cardiac histology following apical right ventricular pacing in patients with congenital atrioventricular block. Pacing Clin Electrophysiol 1999;9:1372–7.
13. Gebauer RA, Tomek V, Kubus P, et al. Differential effects of the site of permanent epicardial pacing on left ventricular synchrony and function in the young: implications for lead placement. Europace 2009;12:1654–9.

14. Tomaske M, Breithardt OA, Bauersfeld U. Preserved cardiac synchrony and function with single-site left ventricular epicardial pacing during mid-term follow-up in paediatric patients. Europace 2009;9: 1168–76.

15. Janousek J, van Geldorp IE, Krupickova, et al. Permanent cardiac pacing in children: choosing the optimal pacing site a multicenter study. Circulation 2013;127:613–23.

16. Cohen MI, Bush DM, Vetter VL, et al. Permanent epicardial pacing in pediatric patients: seventeen years of experience and 1200 outpatient visits. Circulation 2001;21:2585–90.

17. Alhuzaimi A, Roy N, Duncan WJ. Cardiac strangulation from epicardial pacemaker: early recognition and prevention. Cardiol Young 2011;4:471–3.

18. Mah DY, Prakash A, Porras D, et al. Coronary artery compresion from epicardial leads: more common than we think. Heart Rhythm 2018;15:1439–47.

19. Gakenheimer-Smith L, Etheridge S, Niu MC, et al. MRI in pediatric and congenital heart disease patients with CIEDs and epicardial or abandoned leads. Pacing Clin Electrophysiol 2020;8:797–804.

20. Pulver AF, Puchalski MD, Bradley DJ, et al. Safety and imaging quality of MRI in pediatric and adult congenital heart disease patients with pacemakers. Pacing Clin Electrophysiol 2009;4:450–6.

21. Von Bergen NH, Atkins DL, Dick M 2nd, et al. Multicenter study of the effectiveness of implantable cardioverter defibrillators in children and young adults with heart disease. Pediatr Cardiol 2011;32(4): 399–405.

22. Berul CI, Van Hare GF, Kertesz NJ, et al. Results of a multicenter retrospective implantable cardioverter-defibrillator registry of pediatric and congenital heart disease patients. J Am Coll Cardiol 2008;51: 1685–91.

23. Korte T, Köditz H, Niehaus M, et al. High incidence of appropriate and inappropriate ICD therapies in children and adolescents with implantable cardioverter defibrillator. Pacing Clin Electrophysiol 2004;27:924–32.

24. Winkler F, Dave H, Weber R, et al. Long-term outcome of epicardial implantable cardioverter-defibrillator systems in children: results justify its preference in paediatric patients. Europace 2018; 20(9):1484–90.

25. Echt DS, Armstrong K, Schmidt P, et al. Clinical experience, complications, and survival in 70 patients with the automatic implantable cardioverter/defibrillator. Circulation 1985;71(2):289–96.

26. Silka MJ, Kron J, Dunnigan A, et al. Sudden cardiac death and the use of ICDs in pediatric patients. The Pediatric Electrophysiology Society. Circulation 1993;87:800–7.

27. Stephenson EA, Batra AS, Knilans TK, et al. A multicenter experience with novel implantable cardioverter defibrillator configurations in the pediatric and congenital heart disease population. J Cardiovasc Electrophysiol 2006;17:41–6.

28. Berul CI, Triedman JK, Forbess J, et al. Minimally invasive cardioverter defibrillator implantation for children: an animal model and pediatric case report. Pacing Clin Electrophysiol 2001;24:1789–94.

29. Gradaus R, Hammel D, Kotthoff S, et al. Nonthoracotomy implantable cardioverter defibrillator placement in children: use of subcutaneous array leads and abdominally placed implantable cardioverter defibrillators in children. J Cardiovasc Electrophysiol 2001;12:356–60.

30. Bauersfeld U, Tomaske M, Dodge-Khatami A, et al. Initial experience with implantable cardioverter defibrillator systems using epicardial and pleural electrodes in pediatric patients. Ann Thorac Surg 2007; 84(1):303–5.

31. Schneider AE, Burkhart HM, Ackerman MJ, et al. Minimally invasive epicardial implantable cardioverter-defibrillator placement for infants and children: an effective alternative to the transvenous approach. Heart Rhythm 2016;13(9):1905–12.

32. Link MS, Hill SL, Cliff DL, et al. Comparison of frequency of complications of implantable cardioverter-defibrillators in children versus adults. Am J Cardiol 1999;83:263–6.

33. Wilson WR, Greer GE, Grubb BP. Implantable cardioverter defibrillators in children: a single-institutional experience. Ann Thorac Surg 1998;65:775–8.

34. Hsu JC, Marcus GM, Al-Khatib SM, et al. Predictors of an inadequate defibrillation safety margin at ICD implantation: insights from the National Cardiovascular Data Registry. J Am Coll Cardiol 2014;64(3):256–64.

35. Prutkin JM, Wang Y, Escudero CA, et al. Defibrillation safety margin testing in patients with congenital heart disease: results from the NCDR. JACC Clin Electrophysiol 2021;7(9):1145–54.

36. Tan RB, Love C, Halpern D, et al. Rise in defibrillation threshold after postoperative cardiac remodeling in a patient with severe Ebstein's anomaly. HeartRhythm Case Rep 2017;3(6):302–5.

37. Radbill AE, Triedman JK, Berul CI, et al. System survival of nontransvenous implantable cardioverterdefibrillators compared to transvenous implantable cardioverter-defibrillators in pediatric and congenital heart disease patients. Heart Rhythm 2010;7:193–8.

38. Stephenson EA, Cecchin F, Walsh EP, et al. Utility of routine follow up defibrillator threshold testing in congenital heart disease and pediatric populations. J Cardiovasc Electrophysiol 2005;16:69–73.

39. Tomaske M, Pretre R, Rahn M, et al. Epicardial and pleural lead ICD systems in children and adolescents maintain functionality over 5 years. Europace 2008;10:1152–6.

40. Cannon BC, Friedman RA, Fenrich AL, et al. Innovative techniques for placement of implantable

cardioverter-defibrillator leads in patients with limited venous access to theheart. Pacing Clin Electrophysiol 2006;29:181–7.

41. Tonko JB, Blauth C, Rosenthal E, et al. Completely epicardial implantable cardioverter/defibrillator (ICD) and CRT-D systems: a case series and systematic literature review. Pacing Clin Electrophysiol 2021;44(9):1616–30.

42. Love BA, Barrett KS, Alexander ME, et al. Supraventricular arrhythmias in children and young adults with implantable cardioverter defibrillators. J Cardiovasc Electrophysiol 2001;12(10):1097–101.

43. Korte T, Jung W, Spehl S, et al. Incidence of ICD lead related complications during long-term follow-up: comparison of epicardial and endocardial electrode systems. Pacing Clin Electrophysiol 1995; 18(11):2053–61.

44. Silvetti KMS, Drago F, Grutter G, et al. Twenty years of paediatric cardiac pacing: 515 pacemakers and 480 leads implanted in 292 patients. Europace 2006;8:530–6.

45. Mizuno T, Goya M, Hirao K, et al. Implantable epicardial cardioverter-defibrillator-induced localized constrictive pericarditis. Interact Cardiovasc Thorac Surg 2018 Jan 1;26(1):158–60.

46. Goodman LR, Almassi GH, Troup PJ, et al. Complications of automatic implantable cardioverter defibrillators: radiographic, CT, and echocardiographic evaluation. Radiology 1989;170:447–52.

47. Molina JE, Benditt DG, Adler S. Crinkling of epicardial defibrillator patches. A common and serious problem. J Thorac Cardiovasc Surg 1995;110: 258–64.

48. Bowman HC, Shannon KM, Biniwale R, et al. Cardiac implantable device outcomes and lead survival in adult congenital heart disease. Int J Cardiol 2021; 324:52–9.

49. Zipes DP, Roberts D. Results of the international study of the implantable pacemaker cardioverter-defibrillator. A comparison of epicardial and endocardial lead systems. The Pacemaker-Cardioverter-Defibrillator Investigators. Circulation 1995;92(1):59–65.

50. Shah MJ. Implantable cardioverter defibrillator-related complications in the pediatric population. Pacing Clin Electrophysiol 2009;32(Suppl 2):S71–4.

51. Stefanelli CB, Bradley DJ, Leroy S, et al. Implantable cardioverter defibrillator therapy for life-threatening arrhythmias in young patients. J Interv Card Electrophysiol 2002;6(3):235–44.

52. Koopman HM, Vrijmoet-Wiersma CM, Langius JN, et al. Psychological functioning and disease-related quality of life in pediatric patients with an implantable cardioverter defibrillator. Pediatr Cardiol 2012;33:569–75.

53. DeMaso DR, Lauretti A, Spieth L, et al. Psychosocial factors and quality of life in children and adolescents with implantable cardioverter defibrillators. Am J Cardiol 2004;93:582–7.

54. Schneider LM, Wong JJ, Adams R, et al. Posttraumatic stress disorder in pediatric patients with implantable cardioverter-defibrillators and their parents. Heart Rhythm 2022;19(9):1524–9.

55. Kapa S, Rotondi-Trevisan D, Mariano Z, et al. Psychopathology in patients with ICDs over time: results of a prospective study. Pacing Clin Electrophysiol 2010;33(2):198–208.

56. Werner H, Lehmann P, Rüegg A, et al. Health-related quality of life outcomes in pediatric patients with cardiac rhythm devices: a cross-sectional study with case-control comparison. Health Qual Life Outcomes 2019;17(1):152.

Lead Management in Patients with Congenital Heart Disease

Soham Dasgupta, MD[a], Douglas Y. Mah, MD[b],*

KEYWORDS

- Congenital heart disease • Pacemaker • Defibrillator • Pediatrics • Lead • Extraction

KEY POINTS

- Pacing strategy (epicardial vs endocardial, single vs dual chamber) and type of defibrillator implant (single vs dual coil, epicardial vs endocardial vs subcutaneous) is determined by patient size, weight, and operator experience. Decisions must be made with long-term consequences in mind, given the young age in which devices are placed in the pediatric and congenital heart disease population.
- What and how hardware is implanted can affect device longevity. Thoughtful decisions should be made on the type of lead implanted, based on lead durability and ease of extraction.
- Implanters should be mindful of anatomic considerations in patients with congenital heart disease, both in terms of anatomic barriers/obstructions and residual shunts, and also variations in the native conduction system should conduction system pacing be an option.
- Antibiotic and anticoagulation management are vital in reducing device revisions. The use of an antibiotic pouch should be considered for patients with a higher risk of infection (prior device infection or endocarditis, renal dysfunction, hypothyroid, immunocompromised).
- Shared decision making is critical when considering abandoning leads versus extraction and placement of new leads after weighing the risks and benefits of either strategy.

 Video content accompanies this article at http://www.cardiacep.theclinics.com.

INTRODUCTION

Cardiac implantable electronic devices (CIED) are increasingly used in patients with congenital heart disease (CHD). Bradycardias, whether related to sinus node dysfunction (SND) or atrioventricular block (AVB), may necessitate the implantation of a permanent pacemaker while malignant arrhythmias warrant an implantable cardioverter defibrillator (ICD). The inherent complexity of CHD necessitates careful consideration prior to the implantation of a CIED and requires thoughtful decision making with respect to long-term device and lead management in these fragile patients.

While the incidence of post-operative complete AVB is 3% of all congenital cardiac surgeries, approximately 1% will require the implantation of a permanent pacemaker.[1] The incidence of SND is higher in pediatric patients with CHD and varies depending on the type of cardiac lesion/surgery performed.[2] The statistics regarding the incidence of ICD implantation in CHD patients are limited and most data is limited to adults with CHD (ACHD).[3] While a patient with CHD is at higher risk of

---

[a] Division of Pediatric Cardiology, Department of Pediatrics, Norton Children's Hospital, University of Louisville, 231 East Chestnut Street, Louisville, KY 40202, USA; [b] Department of Cardiology, Boston Children's Hospital, Harvard Medical School, 300 Longwood Avenue, Boston, MA 02115, USA
* Corresponding author.
E-mail address: douglas.mah@cardio.chboston.org

Card Electrophysiol Clin 15 (2023) 481–491
https://doi.org/10.1016/j.ccep.2023.06.003

needing a CIED compared to age-matched non-CHD controls, certain lesions are at greater risk including tetralogy of Fallot (TOF), d-transposition of the great arteries (d-TGA), corrected transposition of the great arteries (cc-TGA), single ventricle physiology and lesions involving surgery near the AV node.[4–6]

DETERMINANTS OF PACING/DEFIBRILLATOR STRATEGY BY AGE AND SIZE
Epicardial Versus Endocardial Pacemakers

Unlike adults who almost always get an endocardial CIED system (**Fig. 1**), the pacing strategy (epicardial vs endocardial; single vs dual chamber) in pediatric patients is often dictated by age, size, and weight. While there are recommendations with respect to weight cut-offs for the consideration of epicardial versus endocardial systems[7]; it is also guided by institutional practice/preference and operator experience. The smallest patients up to 15 to 20 kg are usually managed with an epicardial device (see **Fig. 1**). Advantages of epicardial systems include placement during concomitant surgery, avoidance of venous access, and lower thromboembolic risks.[8] Disadvantages include requiring a sternotomy/lateral thoracotomy in a patient not getting concomitant surgery, intrathoracic surgery for future lead revisions, higher incidence of lead failures and longer recovery times.[9–11] Although a transvenous pacing system is feasible under 10 kg,[12] complication rates in smaller children are higher, suggesting that an epicardial system maybe the better alternative.[12] Lead placement in young patients also "starts the clock" on future lead revisions, exposing

patients to the risks of several lead extractions over a lifetime.

Number of Pacing Leads

Single versus dual-chamber pacing is determined by the underlying indication for pacing, cardiac anatomy, and size of the patient. For patients with isolated sinus node dysfunction with no evidence of AV conduction disease, a single chamber atrial pacemaker may be sufficient.[13] In the setting of complete AVB, ventricular pacing alone may be adequate in neonates, infants, and young children as epicardial lead implantation can be accomplished with a small sub-xyphoid incision and fewer leads are likely to leads to fewer complications/interventions over time. This should be weighed against the benefits of atrio-ventricular synchrony, with the addition of an atrial lead reserved for those with significant cardiac symptoms (pre-syncope or syncope) or poor ventricular function.[14,15]

In slightly bigger patients who do not quite meet the criteria for an endocardial system, it may be reasonable to consider a dual chamber system. When an epicardial ventricular lead is being placed, implanting a lead in the left ventricular apex/lateral wall may be beneficial in preventing pacing-induced cardiomyopathy,[16] although caution should be taken in those with complex congenital heart disease.[17]

For endocardial devices, decisions on the number and type of leads implanted should be made with a long-term perspective. A greater number of leads increases the drain on a device's battery, exposing the patient to an increased number of

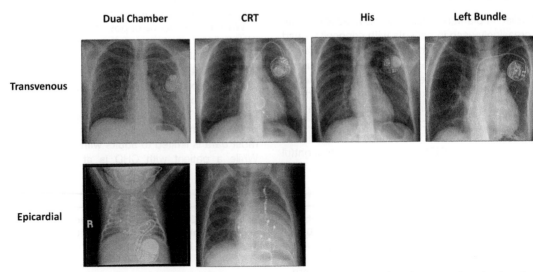

Fig. 1. Representative examples of transvenous and epicardial dual chamber and cardiac resynchronization therapy pacemakers, as well as transvenous examples of His and left bundle area pacing devices.

generator changes, while the leads themselves require revision over time. More leads present means higher risk at the time of extraction.[18] In a large study by Silvetti and colleagues, a dual chamber endocardial system was preferred in patients weighing at least 25 kg.[14] With respect to optimal endocardial pacing strategies in the right ventricle, best left ventricular mechanical performance was achieved by right ventricular septal pacing in the non-apical, mid-superior segments.[19] Newer endocardial "physiologic" pacing strategies include His bundle and left bundle branch pacing.[20,21] Patients who require a high percentage of ventricular pacing and thus who are at a high risk for developing pacemaker-induced cardiomyopathy are individuals who could benefit the most from conduction system pacing (CSP) (see **Fig. 1**).

Another strategy to treat pacing-induced cardiomyopathy is cardiac re-synchronization therapy (CRT). Benefits of CRT in select adult patients have been clearly demonstrated in terms of cardiac remodeling and symptoms.[22] Resynchronization therapy in complete AVB may be achieved either epicardially by placing a second set of ventricular leads or via a traditional endocardial coronary sinus lead, if feasible. Most cases of CRT in the pediatric CHD literature are performed as an upgrade to conventional ventricular pacing because of pacing-associated heart failure, or with a failing systemic right ventricle,[23] though primary biventricular pacing should be considered for select patients. As an example, Hofferberth and colleagues recommended that all patients with cc-TGA who develop complete AVB should undergo primary biventricular pacing.[24] Nevertheless, it should be stressed that CRT in CHD patients is more technically challenging when compared to a structurally normal heart, and often comes with a less predictable response to resynchronization.

Given the challenges of biventricular pacing, there has been an increasing use of CSP.[25] The benefits to CSP in terms of lead management are obvious, with one lead able to perform the function of two, decreasing the amount of hardware placed in younger and smaller patients. The use of the lumenless Medtronic 3830 leads, the most common selection for CSP, also helps with extraction, given their lower profile and high tensile strength.[26] However, patients with CHD often have anatomic abnormalities of the conduction system, making His bundle pacing challenging/ineffective.[20] Left bundle pacing is a newer strategy for physiologic pacing and initial pediatric data is encouraging.[21] The long-term merits of CSP must also be considered in our younger patient population. His bundle

pacing often requires higher pacing outputs, decreasing the battery longevity and increasing the number of generator changes over a lifetime.[27,28] In contrast, left bundle area pacing leads tend to function at pacing outputs in line with conventional RV pacing leads. Their deeper insertion into the septum, however, raises concerns regarding the feasibility of their removal, with extraction data limited to leads less than 2 year old.[29,30]

Implantable Cardioverter Defibrillators

The indications for ICD placement in pediatric and ACHD patients are varied, with the best-studied CHD being TOF.[31–33] It is important to note that ICD generators are larger compared to pacemakers, especially when implantation is considered in a small patient. Additionally, single ventricle physiology and intracardiac shunts may prevent the placement of a transvenous system, necessitating an epicardial or subcutaneous route[34] (**Fig. 2**). Complications associated with epicardial defibrillation leads include an increased risk of lead malfunction and inappropriate shocks.[34] However, this may be the only option for small patients, patients with complex CHD or those with residual intracardiac shunts. While there is increasing evidence for the placement of a subcutaneous ICD system, the generators are significantly larger and lack pacing capabilities (see **Fig. 2**). It is an attractive device in patients who require a "shock box" with no obvious current or future anti-bradycardia or anti-tachycardia pacing needs. While recent results have been promising with respect to efficacy and low rates of complications/lead failures, the experience in CHD patients is lagging.[35,36]

Single coil systems are preferred when an ICD is required, with data showing no significant difference in defibrillation thresholds, first shock efficacy, or all-cause mortality compared to dual coil systems.[37] Dual coil systems are more difficult to extract, with the fibrosis around the SVC coil increasing the risk of mortality if they need to be removed.[38,39] Nevertheless, there are instances in which a dual coil system is required to ensure the defibrillator vector adequately covers the systemic ventricle. For transvenous devices, this approach is more often needed in the setting of right-sided ICDs. Although the literature on these devices is lacking,[40] interactive simulations have shown that right-sided devices have higher defibrillation thresholds,[41] and the presence of a posteriorly located SVC coil can create a voltage gradient that encompasses the heart. Similarly, for epicardial devices, a high-voltage coil located

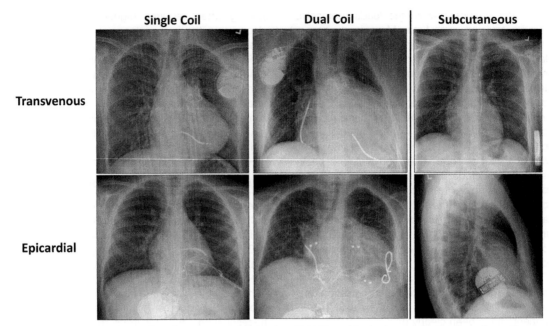

Fig. 2. Representative examples of transvenous and epicardial ICDs, with single and dual coil configurations, as well as an example of a subcutaneous ICD.

posteriorly can provide an adequate defibrillator vector, although attention should also be paid to the location of the abdominal generator. The use of a single coil decreases the amount of hardware implanted and need for future revisions. However, for larger patients, a second coil on the contralateral side of the heart may be required to provide better coverage of the heart.

LEAD FAILURE AND COMPLICATIONS IN PEDIATRIC PATIENTS

The complications related to pacing are higher in CHD patients.[42] While epicardial leads are more prone to fracture and exit block, lead dislodgment and insulation breaks are the primary issues for endocardial systems.[43] Venous occlusion and thromboembolic events are further considerations in transvenous systems.[8]

The advent of steroid-eluting epicardial leads has improved lead longevity.[44,45] This limits the inflammatory response at the electrode-tissue interface resulting in better acute/chronic thresholds.[46] Beaufort-Krol et al. suggested that the longevity of steroid-eluting epicardial leads is similar to conventional endocardial leads; however, this study did not include patients with CHD.[47] Other studies have described the high incidence of epicardial lead failures in CHD at a median time frame of 4.8 years after implantation.[48] A clinical trial evaluated the safety of the Medtronic bipolar Capsure Epi 4968 (Medtronic, Minneapolis USA) bipolar

steroid eluting lead. Adverse events were noted in 9% with the most common event being the loss of capture.[49] Despite these limitations, often this is the only available option for small pediatric patients with CHD.

LEAD CHOICES

Pediatric and CHD patients are often quite young at the time of device implantation. Decisions on the type of hardware implanted can influence the frequency of device revisions and the number of procedures our patients undergo over a lifetime. The type of lead implanted should be decided based on lead longevity and ease of extraction. Additionally, one should be mindful of the risk of venous occlusion given the young age at implant, resultant duration of indwelling leads, and the comparatively smaller cross-sectional area of the systemic veins in pediatric patients.[50] Comparison of lead families commonly used noted similar durability of Medtronic 4076 and Boston Scientific FineLine leads, with the Abbott Tendril leads having a higher incidence of lead failure (7% vs 2%).[51] Caution should be used with FineLine leads, however. Although their construction makes them durable and easy to implant, they are more likely to break at the time of extraction.[52] There is a growing use of Medtronic 3830 SelectSecure leads as the lead of choice for CSP. Given their lumenless and low caliber design, they are less likely to cause atrioventricular valve regurgitation, as well as SVC and innominate vein narrowing.[53] Their increased tensile strength allows them to hold up better under extraction.[26] However, they do have a higher incidence of dislodgement after implant, and their slightly higher capture thresholds can decrease a device's generator battery longevity by approximately 8 months.[54]

With respect to endocardial defibrillator leads, there is variability among manufacturers with respect to lead/device failure.[55] A study evaluating ICD lead reliability demonstrated a lead failure rate of 0.3% per year (median follow up 3.2 years).[56] Dechert and colleagues demonstrated that 33% of pediatric patients with CHD required an ICD revision.[57] The PLEASE study evaluated pediatric and CHD patients with an ICD implanted between 2005 and 2010. The lead failure rate was 14% at a median time of 2 years postimplant. Younger age at lead implantation was associated with higher lead failure rates and older lead age correlated with the need for advanced lead extraction techniques.[58]

PROCEDURAL CHOICES

Choices made during the CIED procedures itself are just as important as the choices made about the type of hardware implanted. The WRAP-IT trial highlighted important modifiable factors to limit the infection risk.[59] It primarily found that the use of an antibiotic envelope can significantly decrease the infection rate over a 1-year follow-up.[60] The patient's anticoagulation strategy can also affect the risk of hematoma and subsequent infection. Warfarin is often continued during procedures in light of the increased infection risk secondary to the use of a heparin bridge.[61] Attempts should be made to keep the INR at the lower end of the therapeutic range. Our institutional practice is to hold antiplatelet medication, if possible, around abdominal generator changes given their risk of bleeding and difficulty placing an adequate pressure bandage. The data on direct oral anticoagulants (DOACs) is less robust, but WRAP-IT did show the use of apixaban had a lower risk of infection compared to other DOACs. If possible, stopping a DOAC the day prior to the procedure and holding it for 72 hours after is ideal. Additionally, a capsulectomy at the time of generator replacement may increase the risk of bleeding and infection.[62,63]

WRAP-IT also found that a chlorhexidine skin prep is preferred over an iodine-based cleanser, and the use of antibiotic wash of the pocket (vs a non-antibiotic wash or no wash) has been shown to decrease the infection risk. WRAP-IT noted an increased risk of infection when using vancomycin (vs cephalosporin). Other studies have noted the benefit of pre-operative antibiotics, but no significant difference in infection rate if antibiotics are continued 2 days post-operatively.[64]

Procedural length has been shown to be an important risk factor for infection, with an increased risk associated with a longer open pocket time. This often reflects case complexity and can be difficult to modify. In our experience, the use of low-temperature electrocautery (PlasmaBlade, Medtronic, Minneapolis USA) may decrease case time, although this was not corroborated in the literature.[65] However, when compared to standard cautery, it can reduce hematoma rates, infection and, importantly, lead injury.

A unique aspect of pediatric implantations is the somatic growth expected after implant. This can make it difficult to determine how much lead length should be left outside the heart and tunneled to an abdominal pocket in epicardial systems, or within the heart in transvenous systems. When placing epicardial leads in young patients, the surgeon must decide how much lead to leave within the mediastinal space, potentially placing the patient at risk for coronary artery compression and strangulation over time,[66] versus too little slack, resulting in tension on the lead and subsequent malfunction.[34] Placing endocardial leads requires a similar balance, with the operator often leaving redundant lead in the right atrium to accommodate future growth. Unfortunately, excess lead can sometimes prolapse through the tricuspid valve or pulmonary valve, leading to worsening valve function, whereas lack of lead redundancy can lead to lead dislodgment and adherence and/or impingement of leaflet mobility.[67–69]

CONSIDERATIONS IN SPECIFIC TYPES OF CONGENITAL HEART DISEASE

Prior to implanting a CIED in a patient with CHD, it is critical to gain detailed knowledge of the underlying anatomy by reviewing the operative notes and advanced imaging if available. Intracardiac shunts need to be carefully evaluated.

Single Ventricles

Single ventricle palliation can make transvenous lead placement challenging. Atrial pacing in the atrio-pulmonary Fontan and the lateral tunnel Fontan may be achievable since there is access to atrial myocardium.[70] Voltage mapping in this setting using an electrophysiology catheter may improve procedural time and precision with respect to lead placement (**Fig. 3**). In patients

RA-PA Fontan   **Lateral Tunnel Fontan**

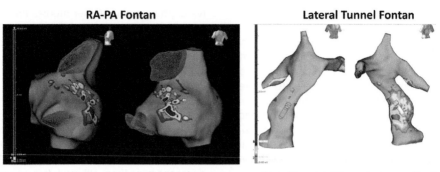

Fig. 3. Voltage maps pre-lead implant to identify isolated areas of healthy atrial tissue in two patients with Fontan palliation.

with extracardiac Fontans, Hemi-Fontan or bidirectional Glenns, placement of an atrial lead can be challenging. There has been the description of techniques for drilling through the pulmonary artery into the roof of the left atrium or directly into the atrium.[65,66] Although endocardial pacing in this patient population may have its advantages, it must be strongly weighed against the risk of thromboembolic events with leads in the systemic circulation.[8,71]

Atrial Switch

Prior to lead implantation in a patient with an atrial switch, an evaluation for baffle stenosis or leaks should take place. Consideration should be given to stenting the baffle prior to lead implantation if required given the high incidence of baffle occlusion after lead placement[72] (**Fig. 4**). Because the natural course of the baffle takes the atrial lead to the lateral atrial wall close to the phrenic nerve, careful evaluation of phrenic capture should be undertaken. It is important to note that the ventricular lead is placed in the smooth-walled left ventricle rather than the naturally trabeculated right ventricle, raising concerns for lead dislodgement.[73] CRT often requires a hybrid epicardial-endocardial approach. With respect to ICD

placement, a high complication rate (27%) has been reported, possibly related to the bulky leads that cross the superior venous baffle.[74]

LEAD EXTRACTION

Guidelines have been published on lead management in the pediatric and congenital heart population,[75] with clear recommendations on the removal of leads in the setting of infection/significant obstruction. However, the best course of action for leads that require replacement but are not infected or causing significant venous obstruction remains unclear. The guidelines state, "Lead removal may be considered for patients … taking into account the number of leads present, patient age, size, venous capacitance, and potential for vascular occlusion." Although abandoning leads does defer the risk of extraction for the present procedure, long-term thinking is needed, and this is often a shared decision between patient and provider. Abandoned leads may require removal in the future, with each year retained increasing the risk for a subsequent extraction. The data on abandoning versus extracting leads is limited. In adults, there is data comparing elderly patients (median age of 78 years) who have had their leads

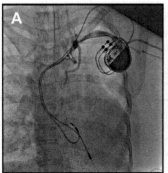
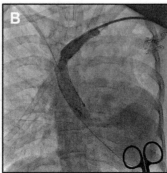
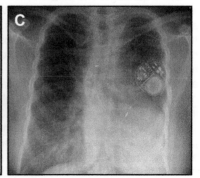

Fig. 4. Example of patient with an atrial switch. Original leads resulted in innominate and SVC obstruction (*A*). Leads were extracted and obstruction was dilated and stented (*B*) before a new system was placed (*C*).

abandoned versus extracted.[76] This did not note any difference in 5-year mortality between the two groups, although there was a lower incidence of infection in those in whom leads were extracted. This is difficult to extrapolate for the much younger population managed by pediatric and congenital electrophysiologists, with patients expected to live for many decades beyond what has been studied.

Of note, there have been some who advocate for prophylactic removal of leads – taking out leads that are still functional – at the time of generator changes. As older leads are harder to remove, the argument is to remove leads before they have time to build up dense adhesions.[77] This would ideally limit the risk of extractions in the future, while also reducing lead revisions between generator changes. Although the proactive approach is appealing, there is literature comparing patients whose leads were replaced at the time of generator change versus those in whom leads were reused.[78] This showed that reused leads were less likely to fail compared to new leads placed at the time of generator change. Thus, leads that have "proven" themselves over the course of a generator's battery life are more likely to last longer. This study should give us pause when deciding on taking out leads that are still functional.

The data on whether lead extraction is different in the pediatric and CHD population is conflicting.[79,80] It is reasonable to assume that the procedure may be complicated by the underlying anatomy and prior surgical repairs as well as the age of the patient at the time of lead implant and extraction. There has also been an increasing awareness of the effect of transvenous leads on tricuspid valve function, especially in the setting of lead extractions. Tricuspid valve dysfunction is often underdiagnosed by transthoracic echocardiography.[69] When applied to patients undergoing lead extraction, studies have found that the degree of tricuspid regurgitation significantly increases in greater than 10% of patients after lead removal,[81,82] although less than 0.5% required surgical intervention. In contrast, the risk for tricuspid and subpulmonary valve injury in children and patients with CHD may be much higher, with one study noting significant regurgitation post-extraction in 3% of patients. Although lead age plays a large role in the risk for tricuspid injury, the patient's age at implant may also be a factor, with leads placed prior to puberty requiring an increased need for complex extraction (**Fig. 5**).[68]

Studies in the adult population have also noted that younger patients (<40 years of age) may need more advanced extraction techniques.[83,84] Techniques for lead extraction are beyond the

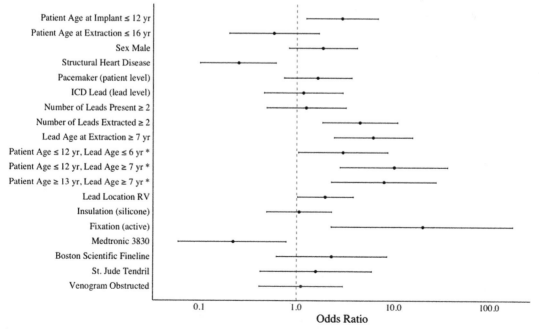

Fig. 5. Univariate risk factors for complex extraction (use of powered sheaths) in the pediatric and congenital heart disease population. * patient age at lead implantation, lead age at extraction. (*From* Pham TDN, Cecchin F, O'Leary E, et al. Lead Extraction at a Pediatric/Congenital Heart Disease Center: The Importance of Patient Age at Implant. JACC Clin Electrophysiol. 2022;8(3):343-353; with permission.)

scope of this review, but it should be highlighted that operators should be prepared for femoral extraction in young patients. The use of femoral extraction allows for leads to be removed after they fracture following a superior approach, while snaring of the leads ahead of time can allow for better traction of the leads, making it safer and easier for powered sheaths to traverse obstructed vessels or tight turns (Videos 1 and 2).

To improve the safety and efficacy of extraction, there has been an increased focus on imaging techniques to guide preprocedural planning, and intraoperative decision making. We have been increasingly employing transesophageal echocardiography during lead extractions. Not only can they better assess the degree of tricuspid regurgitation post-extraction, but it has been shown to be useful in identifying both lead binding sites and excess lead loops bound to important structures.[85] Cardiac computed tomography (CT) has been shown to be helpful in assessing the degree of fibrosis surrounding a lead and whether it is embedded within or located outside a vessel.[86–88] As the degree of adhesions affects procedural time, the need for powered sheaths, and more complex extraction techniques, imaging can help not only with procedural planning, but also with patient counseling. Shared decision making is important in deciding how aggressive to be with removing leads.

CLINICS CARE POINTS

- The type of CIED implanted is dictated by patient size and anatomy with the consideration of the patient's need for long-term lead management.

- Although an endocardial pacing system placement is feasible in patients under 10 kg, complication rates suggest that an epicardial system maybe a better alternative.

- Cardiac resynchronization therapy can be considered in patients who require a high percentage of ventricular pacing. Conduction system pacing may be a suitable alternative but long-term follow-up is lacking.

- Epicardial ICDs may be the only option for small patients and patients with single ventricles or residual intracardiac shunts, although data demonstrates shorter survival of these systems. Some patients with suitable QRS morphologies may screen in for subcutaneous ICDs, but the size of the generator limits patient selection.

- The addition of steroid elution has improved epicardial lead longevity.

- Lumenless pacing leads are less likely to cause atrioventricular valve regurgitation and superior vena caval/innominate vein narrowing, and may hold up better during extraction.

- Use of an antibiotic envelope during the procedure and peri-operative anticoagulation strategies can have a significant impact on the rate of device-related infections.

- Shared decision making is recommended when discussing abandoning leads versus extraction. Removal and replacement of functional pacing leads during generator changes has not been shown to be an effective long-term strategy.

DISCLOSURE

The authors have nothing to disclose.

SUPPLEMENTARY DATA

Supplementary data related to this article can be found online at https://doi.org/10.1016/j.ccep.2023.06.003.

REFERENCES

1. Duong SQ, Shi Y, Giacone H, et al. Criteria for early pacemaker implantation in patients with postoperative heart block after congenital heart surgery. Circ Arrhythm Electrophysiol 2022;15:e011145.
2. Greenwood RD, Rosenthal A, Sloss LJ, et al. Sick sinus syndrome after surgery for congenital heart disease. Circulation 1975;52:208–13.
3. Vehmeijer JT, Brouwer TF, Limpens J, et al. Implantable cardioverter-defibrillators in adults with congenital heart disease: a systematic review and meta-analysis. Eur Heart J 2016;37:1439–48.
4. Czosek RJ, Anderson J, Khoury PR, et al. Utility of ambulatory monitoring in patients with congenital heart disease. Am J Cardiol 2013;111:723–30.
5. Gelatt M, Hamilton RM, McCrindle BW, et al. Arrhythmia and mortality after the Mustard procedure: a 30-year single-center experience. J Am Coll Cardiol 1997;29:194–201.
6. Rutledge JM, Nihill MR, Fraser CD, et al. Outcome of 121 patients with congenitally corrected transposition of the great arteries. Pediatr Cardiol 2002;23: 137–45.
7. Brugada J, Blom N, Sarquella-Brugada G, et al. Pharmacological and non-pharmacological therapy for arrhythmias in the pediatric population: EHRA

and AEPC-Arrhythmia Working Group joint consensus statement. Europace 2013;15:1337–82.

8. Khairy P, Landzberg MJ, Gatzoulis MA, et al. Transvenous pacing leads and systemic thromboemboli in patients with intracardiac shunts: a multicenter study. Circulation 2006;113:2391–7.

9. Silvetti MS, Drago F, Di Carlo D, et al. Cardiac pacing in paediatric patients with congenital heart defects: transvenous or epicardial? Europace 2013; 15:1280–6.

10. Fortescue EB, Berul CI, Cecchin F, et al. Patient, procedural, and hardware factors associated with pacemaker lead failures in pediatrics and congenital heart disease. Heart Rhythm 2004;1: 150–9.

11. Sachweh JS, Vazquez-Jimenez JF, Schondube FA, et al. Twenty years experience with pediatric pacing: epicardial and transvenous stimulation. Eur J Cardio Thorac Surg 2000;17:455–61.

12. Vos LM, Kammeraad JAE, Freund MW, et al. Long-term outcome of transvenous pacemaker implantation in infants: a retrospective cohort study. Europace 2017;19:581–7.

13. Gillette PC, Shannon C, Garson A Jr, et al. Pacemaker treatment of sick sinus syndrome in children. J Am Coll Cardiol 1983;1:1325–9.

14. Silvetti MS, Drago F, Grutter G, et al. Twenty years of paediatric cardiac pacing: 515 pacemakers and 480 leads implanted in 292 patients. Europace 2006;8:530–6.

15. Chaouki AS, Spar DS, Khoury PR, et al. Risk factors for complications in the implantation of epicardial pacemakers in neonates and infants. Heart Rhythm 2017;14:206–10.

16. Janousek J, van Geldorp IE, Krupickova S, et al. Permanent cardiac pacing in children: choosing the optimal pacing site: a multicenter study. Circulation 2013;127:613–23.

17. Koubsky K, Kovanda J, Lozek M, et al. Multisite pacing for heart failure associated with left ventricular apical pacing in congenital heart disease. JACC Clin Electrophysiol 2022;8:1060–4.

18. Agarwal SK, Kamireddy S, Nemec J, et al. Predictors of complications of endovascular chronic lead extractions from pacemakers and defibrillators: a single-operator experience. J Cardiovasc Electrophysiol 2009;20:171–5.

19. Vancura V, Wichterle D, Melenovsky V, et al. Assessment of optimal right ventricular pacing site using invasive measurement of left ventricular systolic and diastolic function. Europace 2013;15:1482–90.

20. Lyon S, Dandamudi G, Kean AC. Permanent His-bundle pacing in pediatrics and congenital heart disease. J Innov Card Rhythm Manag 2020;11: 4005–12.

21. Jimenez E, Zaban N, Sharma N, et al. His bundle and left bundle pacing in pediatrics and congenital heart disease: a single center experience. Pediatr Cardiol 2020;41:1425–31.

22. Turschner O, Ritscher G, Simon H, et al. Criteria for patient selection in cardiac resynchronization therapy. Future Cardiol 2010;6:871–80.

23. Janousek J. Cardiac resynchronisation in congenital heart disease. Heart 2009;95:940–7.

24. Hofferberth SC, Alexander ME, Mah DY, et al. Impact of pacing on systemic ventricular function in L-transposition of the great arteries. J Thorac Cardiovasc Surg 2016;151:131–8.

25. Vijayaraman P, Zalavadia D, Haseeb A, et al. Clinical outcomes of conduction system pacing compared to biventricular pacing in patients requiring cardiac resynchronization therapy. Heart Rhythm 2022;19: 1263–71.

26. Shepherd E, Stuart G, Martin R, et al. Extraction of SelectSecure leads compared to conventional pacing leads in patients with congenital heart disease and congenital atrioventricular block. Heart Rhythm 2015;12:1227–32.

27. Beer D, Subzposh FA, Colburn S, et al. His bundle pacing capture threshold stability during long-term follow-up and correlation with lead slack. Europace 2021;23:757–66.

28. Vijayaraman P, Naperkowski A, Subzposh FA, et al. Permanent His-bundle pacing: long-term lead performance and clinical outcomes. Heart Rhythm 2018;15:696–702.

29. Chen X, Wei L, Bai J, et al. Procedure-related complications of left bundle branch pacing: a single-center experience. Front Cardiovasc Med 2021;8: 645947.

30. Vijayaraman P. Extraction of left bundle branch pacing lead. JACC Clin Electrophysiol 2020;6:903–4.

31. Epstein AE, Dimarco JP, Ellenbogen KA, et al. ACC/AHA/HRS 2008 Guidelines for device-based therapy of cardiac rhythm abnormalities. Heart Rhythm 2008;5:e1–62.

32. Khairy P, Harris L, Landzberg MJ, et al. Implantable cardioverter-defibrillators in tetralogy of Fallot. Circulation 2008;117:363–70.

33. Atallah J, Gonzalez Corcia MC, Walsh EP, et al. Ventricular arrhythmia and life-threatening events in patients with repaired tetralogy of Fallot. Am J Cardiol 2020;132:126–32.

34. Radbill AE, Triedman JK, Berul CI, et al. System survival of nontransvenous implantable cardioverter-defibrillators compared to transvenous implantable cardioverter-defibrillators in pediatric and congenital heart disease patients. Heart Rhythm 2010;7:193–8.

35. Lambiase PD, Theuns DA, Murgatroyd F, et al. Subcutaneous implantable cardioverter-defibrillators: long-term results of the EFFORTLESS study. Eur Heart J 2022;43:2037–50.

36. Kobe J, Reinke F, Meyer C, et al. Implantation and follow-up of totally subcutaneous versus conventional

implantable cardioverter-defibrillators: a multicenter case-control study. Heart Rhythm 2013;10:29–36.

37. Sunderland N, Kaura A, Murgatroyd F, et al. Outcomes with single-coil versus dual-coil implantable cardioverter defibrillators: a meta-analysis. Europace 2018;20:e21–9.

38. Epstein LM, Love CJ, Wilkoff BL, et al. Superior vena cava defibrillator coils make transvenous lead extraction more challenging and riskier. J Am Coll Cardiol 2013;61:987–9.

39. Segreti L, Di Cori A, Soldati E, et al. Major predictors of fibrous adherences in transvenous implantable cardioverter-defibrillator lead extraction. Heart Rhythm 2014;11:2196–201.

40. Pham TDN, Valente AM, Mayer JE, et al. Implanted pacemaker and cardioverter-defibrillator in a patient with ectopia cordis. HeartRhythm Case Rep 2020;6: 110–3.

41. Jolley M, Stinstra J, Pieper S, et al. A computer modeling tool for comparing novel ICD electrode orientations in children and adults. Heart Rhythm 2008; 5:565–72.

42. McLeod CJ, Attenhofer Jost CH, Warnes CA, et al. Epicardial versus endocardial permanent pacing in adults with congenital heart disease. J Interv Card Electrophysiol 2010;28:235–43.

43. Lotfy W, Hegazy R, AbdElAziz O, et al. Permanent cardiac pacing in pediatric patients. Pediatr Cardiol 2013;34:273–80.

44. Gillette PC, Zeigler V, Bradham GB, et al. Pediatric transvenous pacing: a concern for venous thrombosis? Pacing Clin Electrophysiol 1988;11:1935–9.

45. Wiegand UK, Potratz J, Bonnemeier H, et al. Long-term superiority of steroid elution in atrial active fixation platinum leads. Pacing Clin Electrophysiol 2000;23:1003–9.

46. Mond HG, Stokes KB. The electrode-tissue interface: the revolutionary role of steroid elution. Pacing Clin Electrophysiol 1992;15:95–107.

47. Beaufort-Krol GC, Mulder H, Nagelkerke D, et al. Comparison of longevity, pacing, and sensing characteristics of steroid-eluting epicardial versus conventional endocardial pacing leads in children. J Thorac Cardiovasc Surg 1999;117:523–8.

48. Post MC, Budts W, Van de Bruaene A, et al. Failure of epicardial pacing leads in congenital heart disease: not uncommon and difficult to predict. Neth Heart J 2011;19:331–5.

49. Inc., M. Model 4968 Capture Epi Steroid-Eluting Bipolar Epicardial Pacing Lead Post-approval Study. ClinicalTrials.gov. 2014;NCT01076361.

50. Silvetti MS, Drago F, De Santis A, et al. Single-centre experience on endocardial and epicardial pacemaker system function in neonates and infants. Europace 2007;9:426–31.

51. El-Chami MF, Rao B, Shah AD, et al. Long-term performance of a pacing lead family: a single-center experience. Heart Rhythm 2019;16:572–8.

52. Morita J, Yamaji K, Nagashima M, et al. Predictors of lead break during transvenous lead extraction. J Arrhythm 2021;37:645–52.

53. Bharmanee A, Zelin K, Sanil Y, et al. Comparative chronic valve and venous effects of lumenless versus stylet-delivered pacing leads in patients with and without congenital heart. Pacing Clin Electrophysiol 2015;38:1343–50.

54. Moak JP, Law IH, LaPage MJ, et al. Comparison of the Medtronic SelectSecure and conventional pacing leads: long-term follow-up in a multicenter pediatric and congenital cohort. Pacing Clin Electrophysiol 2019;42:356–65.

55. Shafat T, Baumfeld Y, Novack V, et al. Significant differences in the expected versus observed longevity of implantable cardioverter defibrillators (ICDs). Clin Res Cardiol 2013;102:43–9.

56. Kramer DB, Hatfield LA, McGriff D, et al. Transvenous implantable cardioverter-defibrillator lead reliability: implications for postmarket surveillance. J Am Heart Assoc 2015;4:e001672.

57. Dechert BE, Bradley DJ, Serwer GA, et al. Implantable cardioverter defibrillator outcomes in pediatric and congenital heart disease: time to system revision. Pacing Clin Electrophysiol 2016;39:703–8.

58. Atallah J, Erickson CC, Cecchin F, et al. Multi-institutional study of implantable defibrillator lead performance in children and young adults: results of the Pediatric Lead Extractability and Survival Evaluation (PLEASE) study. Circulation 2013;127:2393–402.

59. Tarakji KG, Krahn AD, Poole JE, et al. Risk factors for CIED infection after secondary procedures: insights from the WRAP-IT trial. JACC Clin Electrophysiol 2022;8:101–11.

60. Tarakji KG, Mittal S, Kennergren C, et al. Antibacterial envelope to prevent cardiac implantable device infection. N Engl J Med 2019;380:1895–905.

61. Birnie DH, Healey JS, Wells GA, et al. Pacemaker or defibrillator surgery without interruption of anticoagulation. N Engl J Med 2013;368:2084–93.

62. Goldenberg GR, Barsheshet A, Bishara J, et al. Effect of fibrotic capsule debridement during generator replacement on cardiac implantable electronic device infection risk. J Interv Card Electrophysiol 2020;58:113–8.

63. Lakkireddy D, Pillarisetti J, Atkins D, et al. IMpact of pocKet rEvision on the rate of InfecTion and other CompLications in patients rEquiring pocket mAnipulation for generator replacement and/or lead replacement or revisioN (MAKE IT CLEAN): a prospective randomized study. Heart Rhythm 2015;12: 950–6.

64. Krahn AD, Longtin Y, Philippon F, et al. Prevention of arrhythmia device infection trial: the PADIT trial. J Am Coll Cardiol 2018;72:3098–109.

65. Mittal S, Wilkoff BL, Poole JE, et al. Low-temperature electrocautery reduces adverse effects from

secondary cardiac implantable electronic device procedures: insights from the WRAP-IT trial. Heart Rhythm 2021;18:1142–50.

66. Mah DY, Prakash A, Porras D, et al. Coronary artery compression from epicardial leads: more common than we think. Heart Rhythm 2018;15:1439–47.

67. Berul CI, Villafane J, Atkins DL, et al. Pacemaker lead prolapse through the pulmonary valve in children. Pacing Clin Electrophysiol 2007;30: 1183–9.

68. Pham TDN, Cecchin F, O'Leary E, et al. Lead extraction at a pediatric/congenital heart disease center: the importance of patient age at implant. JACC Clin Electrophysiol 2022;8:343–53.

69. Lin G, Nishimura RA, Connolly HM, et al. Severe symptomatic tricuspid valve regurgitation due to permanent pacemaker or implantable cardioverter-defibrillator leads. J Am Coll Cardiol 2005;45: 1672–5.

70. Takahashi K, Cecchin F, Fortescue E, et al. Permanent atrial pacing lead implant route after Fontan operation. Pacing Clin Electrophysiol 2009;32: 779–85.

71. Assaad IE, Pastor T, O'Leary E, et al. Atrial pacing in Fontan patients: the effect of transvenous lead on clot burden. Heart Rhythm 2021;18:1860–7.

72. Khairy P, Landzberg MJ, Lambert J, et al. Long-term outcomes after the atrial switch for surgical correction of transposition: a meta-analysis comparing the Mustard and Senning procedures. Cardiol Young 2004;14:284–92.

73. Konings TC, Dekkers LR, Groenink M, et al. Transvenous pacing after the Mustard procedure: considering the complications. Neth Heart J 2007;15: 387–9.

74. Bouzeman A, Marijon E, de Guillebon M, et al. Implantable cardiac defibrillator among adults with transposition of the great arteries and atrial switch operation: case series and review of literature. Int J Cardiol 2014;177:301–6.

75. Writing Committee M, Shah MJ, Silka MJ, et al. 2021 PACES expert consensus statement on the indications and management of cardiovascular implantable electronic devices in pediatric patients. Heart Rhythm 2021;18:1888–924.

76. Pokorney SD, Mi X, Lewis RK, et al. Outcomes associated with extraction versus capping and abandoning pacing and defibrillator leads. Circulation 2017; 136:1387–95.

77. Keiler J, Schulze M, Dreger R, et al. Quantitative and qualitative assessment of adhesive thrombo-fibrotic lead encapsulations (TFLE) of pacemaker and ICD leads in arrhythmia patients-A post mortem study. Front Cardiovasc Med 2020;7:602179.

78. Whitehill RD, Chandler SF, DeWitt E, et al. Lead age as a predictor for failure in pediatrics and congenital heart disease. Pacing Clin Electrophysiol 2021;44: 586–94.

79. McCanta AC, Kong MH, Carboni MP, et al. Laser lead extraction in congenital heart disease: a case-controlled study. Pacing Clin Electrophysiol 2013; 36:372–80.

80. Cecchin F, Atallah J, Walsh EP, et al. Lead extraction in pediatric and congenital heart disease patients. Circ Arrhythm Electrophysiol 2010;3:437–44.

81. Park SJ, Gentry JL 3rd, Varma N, et al. Transvenous extraction of pacemaker and defibrillator leads and the risk of tricuspid valve regurgitation. JACC Clin Electrophysiol 2018;4:1421–8.

82. Coffey JO, Sager SJ, Gangireddy S, et al. The impact of transvenous lead extraction on tricuspid valve function. Pacing Clin Electrophysiol 2014;37: 19–24.

83. El-Chami MF, Merchant FM, Waheed A, et al. Predictors and outcomes of lead extraction requiring a bailout femoral approach: data from 2 high-volume centers. Heart Rhythm 2017;14:548–52.

84. El-Chami MF, Sayegh MN, Patel A, et al. Outcomes of lead extraction in young adults. Heart Rhythm 2017;14:537–40.

85. Nowosielecka D, Jachec W, Polewczyk A, et al. The role of transesophageal echocardiography in predicting technical problems and complications of transvenous lead extractions procedures. Clin Cardiol 2021;44:1233–42.

86. Svennberg E, Jacobs K, McVeigh E, et al. Computed tomography-guided risk assessment in percutaneous lead extraction. JACC Clin Electrophysiol 2019;5:1439–46.

87. Patel D, Vatterott P, Piccini J, et al. Prospective evaluation of the correlation between gated cardiac computed tomography detected vascular fibrosis and ease of transvenous lead extraction. Circ Arrhythm Electrophysiol 2022;15:e010779.

88. Patel D, Sripariwuth A, Abozeed M, et al. Lead location as assessed on cardiac computed tomography and difficulty of percutaneous transvenous extraction. JACC Clin Electrophysiol 2019;5:1432–8.

Prediction of Sudden Death Risk in Patients with Congenital Heart Diseases

Rohan Kumthekar, MD[a,b], Gregory Webster, MD, MPH[c],*

KEYWORDS

- Congenital heart disease • Sudden death • Risk stratification • Arrhythmia • Defibrillator • Pediatric

KEY POINTS

- The risk of sudden death in congenital heart disease (CHD) is at least 20 times higher than the normal population.
- Six major risk factors for sudden death include anatomy, symptoms, systemic ventricular function, atrial arrhythmias, ventricular arrhythmias, and pulmonary hypertension.
- Despite advances in ablation, implantable cardioverter defibrillator (ICD) therapy remains the mainstay of sudden death prevention.
- New technologies in ICDs continue to be adapted to the CHD population, but devices designed for pediatric use are not yet readily available.

NATURE OF THE PROBLEM

In 2023, the field of congenital heart disease (CHD) remains frustratingly far away from the optimal triad of risk prevention: accurate stratification of risk, effective risk modifiers (medical, surgical, behavioral, or environmental), and comprehensive data to weigh the advantages and disadvantages of each modification. For this article, we will define CHD as hearts with anatomic lesions resulting in abnormal blood course or abnormal pressure/volume loading and exclude congenital and genetic lesions such as cardiomyopathy and hyperlipidemia.

Highly modifiable risk factors for sudden death include ventricular pre-excitation and major coronary anomalies. However, the prevalence of these highly modifiable risk factors is low. Other risk factors, such as moderate-to-severe systolic dysfunction of the systemic ventricle, are harder to reverse. The primary goal of risk stratification is to identify higher risk characteristics for each patient and to identify the most effective way to modify risk that is acceptable to the patient.

Prevalence

Mortality from CHD has been on the decline for half a century, falling precipitously between 1995 and 2005.[1] However, sudden death still occurs approximately 20 to 30 times as frequently in CHD as it does in the general population[2] and accounts for approximately 25% of deaths in CHD (**Fig. 1**). The epidemiologic risk of sudden death in CHD is heterogeneous, and data collection regarding the risk of sudden death in patients with CHD is imperfect. Even in the best studies, the relative rarity of CHD means that patients with diverse physiologies will be lumped together. Many studies trade specificity for power, allowing us to identify sudden death risk factors, but limiting the specificity of those factors.[3,4] If perioperative mortality is excluded, adults with CHD have a higher incidence of sudden death than younger

a Division of Cardiology, Nationwide Children's Hospital, 700 Children's Drive, Columbus, OH 43205, USA;
b Department of Pediatrics, The Ohio State University College of Medicine, 370 W. 9th Avenue, Columbus, OH, USA; c Division of Cardiology, Ann & Robert H. Lurie Children's Hospital of Chicago, Northwestern University Feinberg School of Medicine, 225 East Chicago Avenue, Box 21, Chicago, IL 60611, USA
* Corresponding author.
E-mail address: rgwebster@luriechildrens.org

Card Electrophysiol Clin 15 (2023) 493–503
https://doi.org/10.1016/j.ccep.2023.07.004

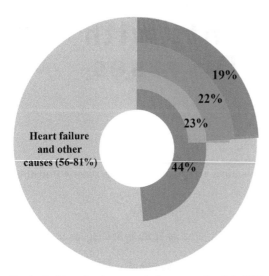

19%

22%

23%

Heart failure
and other
causes (56-81%)

44%

Fig. 1. Sudden death accounts for approximately 25% of mortality in congenital heart disease (CHD). The circle represents all deaths in congenital heart disease. Colored stripes represent the percentage of sudden death in 4 studies: purple (6933 patients),[66] pink (8595 patients),[67] light blue (2596 patients),[68] and dark blue (936 patients).[4] Two of these sampled data from the CONgenital CORvitia(CONCOR) registry.[66,67] The gray background indicates death from all other causes, predominantly heart failure.

CHD patients. The nuances of the age-risk relationship remain imperfectly described. Some studies suggest that patientswith severe CHD face the apex of sudden death risk during their 20s and 30s and that patients with less severe disease have a smaller sudden death peak in their 50s, but survivorship bias colors these conclusions.[5–7]

Many studies on high-risk CHD have occurred in tertiary care centers, with resultant referral bias and survivorship bias. In addition, sudden death is often inaccurately modeled as an arrhythmia event. Sudden death without primary bradycardia or tachyarrhythmias may account for 10% to 25% of sudden deaths.[8] Thus, while ICDs are a major life-saving technology, they are not effective in all life-threatening scenarios.

Specific Risk Factors

While many individual risk factors have merited publication, we focus on 6 major risk factors for sudden death (**Fig. 2**).

Anatomic Substrate and Surgical Repair

The initial risk assessment depends on anatomic substrate. The highest risk of sudden death occurs in transposition substrates, Ebstein anomaly of the tricuspid valve, single ventricle physiology, and tetralogy of Fallot (ToF). The mid-tier of risk includes aortic valve abnormalities, atrioventricular septal defects, and severe aortic coarctation.[9] With rare exceptions, most other surgically repaired or palliated lesions are in a lower risk tier.

Anatomy matters, but published lesion-specific sudden death rates are still approximations. For example, population studies report a lower rate of sudden death among age-matched ToF patients compared to single ventricles.[9] Despite these overall trends, a recent expert committee estimated the annualized sudden death rate in ToF as 0.9% to 1.5% per year.[2] This is 5-fold to 10-fold higher than the estimate of the ventricular tachycardia or sudden death in Fontan palliations (0.15%–0.2% per year) by an equally experienced committee of single ventricle experts.[10] Thus, there is mismatch between assessments of relative risk and absolute risk between anatomic lesions.

Risk can also depend on surgical approach. For example, long-term risks in patients with [S,D,D] transposition who were palliated with an atrial switch differ from patients palliated with an arterial switch. However, even when the palliation choices are not so starkly different, small details of anatomic repair such as perfusion times, coronary artery repositioning, and anatomic approach likely influence long-term outcomes.

Systolic Dysfunction of the Systemic Ventricle

The single best-documented mortality risk factor in CHD is systolic dysfunction of the systemic ventricle. Its contribution to CHD risk has been demonstrated in over a dozen studies of various anatomic substrates; a typical finding is a hazard ratio of 29 in favor of sudden death among patients with severe dysfunction of the systemic ventricle (<35%) compared to all other assessments of systolic ventricular function.[4] Routine assessment of ventricular systolic function, whether by echocardiography or cross-sectional imaging, is a mandatory component of risk assessment in CHD.

Several studies have demonstrated a relationship between diastolic dysfunction and death/transplant. However, in a study of 556 patients with ToF using ventricular tachycardia as an outcome measure, the positive predictive value of diastolic dysfunction assessed by echocardiography was 29%, compared to a negative predictive value of 90%.[11] Thus, normal diastolic parameters are a marker of safety, but the presence of diastolic dysfunction does not imply that ventricular tachycardia is imminent, at least in 1 anatomic substrate. Data in other substrates remain scant.

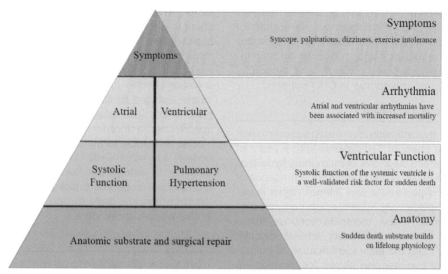

Fig. 2. Six risk factors for sudden death in congenital heart disease.

Symptoms

Syncope remains the most important symptom affecting risk stratification. The presence of unexplained syncope with a potentially arrhythmic substrate in CHD is a Class IIA or IIB indication for ICD.[12] One ongoing question in electrophysiology (EP) practice remains when to place an implantable loop recorder (ILR). Some authors have advocated using ILRs in asymptomatic patients; others have restricted the use to patients with symptoms. The selection process for ILR placement yields different rates of arrhythmia burden (27% to 60% in CHD studies published in the last 5 years)[13–16] and use of an ILR in this population remains guided by individual differences in physician judgment. We anticipate that the threshold for ILR implantation will continue to change in the next several years.

Ventricular Arrhythmia

Risk stratification with programmed ventricular stimulation has been incorporated into ICD guidelines. This technique has been most thoroughly evaluated in ToF, in which a positive ventricular stimulation study is associated with a higher risk of a sudden death event. Two studies demonstrate that this approach can be useful for Bayesian analysis, but that a positive ventricular stimulation study does not determine patient outcomes in isolation. In ToF, ventricular arrhythmias were induced during programmed stimulation in approximately 25% of the patients[17,18]; however, the positive predictive value of inducible arrhythmia was only 24% during a mean follow-up of 4.3 years.[18] While an event rate of approximately 5%/year is useful in guiding patient-centered discussions about ICDs, it is not

necessarily an indication for device placement in isolation.

Ambulatory monitors can screen for bradycardia and atrial arrhythmias, but they are less effective in evaluating ventricular arrhythmias and sudden death risk. A 10-year study in CHD reported non-sustained ventricular tachycardia in 8% of all Holter monitors, with no difference in the subsequent rate of sudden cardiac events between groups with and without non-sustained ventricular tachycardia.[19] This study reinforces other data that non-sustained ventricular tachycardia on Holter monitoring is not sufficient as an isolated feature to demand immediate intervention. Exercise tests are not typically used as a primary screening tool for sudden death risk in CHD, except in selected populations with exercise-related symptoms.

Atrial Arrhythmia

Atrial arrhythmias are an important yet incompletely understood risk factor for sudden death. In two examples, atrial arrhythmia risk in CHD was evaluated in 38,428 adults with CHD, of whom 5812 had atrial arrhythmias.[3] The hazard ratio for any serious adverse event was 2.5 and the hazard ratio for mortality was 1.5. A separate study demonstrated that the prevalence of atrial arrhythmias varies by disease substrate (5% in adults with ventricular septal defects compared to 33% of adults with Ebstein anomaly, for example).[3] While it is possible that the mortality association for atrial arrhythmias is not causative (atrial arrhythmia may be an effect of other physiologic problems, rather than causing those problems), several studies, including recent single ventricle work,[20] reinforce that atrial arrhythmias co-segregate with mortality in adults with CHD. The frequency and modality of screening for atrial arrhythmias should be individualized to the patient's age, substrate, and symptoms, but we advocate for early and thoughtful control of atrial arrhythmias in CHD patients.

Pulmonary Hypertension

Pulmonary hypertension is an independent marker of risk. In a study of 310 patients with 6 years of follow-up after a diagnosis of pulmonary hypertension, the mortality hazard ratio for the presence of pulmonary hypertension was 3 times higher in patients with pulmonary hypertension compared to those without.[21] New therapies continue to be developed to lower pulmonary arterial vascular resistance[22] and the early identification of pulmonary arterial hypertension allows for assessment of anatomic lesions and initiation of early palliative or interventional therapy. Pulmonary hypertension remains a rare, but important risk factor for sudden death and it is an area where new therapies may provide additional strategies to alter the long-term risk of sudden death.

Tetralogy of Fallot (ToF)

The risk of ventricular arrhythmia and sudden death has been studied more comprehensively in ToF than in any other CHD lesion. Many of the data to support the aforementioned 6 primary risk factors have been derived from studies dominated by patients with ToF. A recent, well-executed meta-analysis of ToF also identified lesion-specific risk

factors (**Table 1**).[23] For example, prior palliative shunt is a risk factor for mortality in ToF, but this represents a very specific surgical approach to repair. Data on palliative shunts in ToF cannot be easily extrapolated to lesions where a staged shunt palliation is rarely (or never) indicated or to lesions where a staged palliative shunt is inevitable in the current era. Ultimately, there are likely lesion-specific risk factors for each type of CHD. Large studies amenable to meta-analysis are not on the horizon for most CHD. Clinicians will need to continue to extrapolate risk from available data and use our collective imaginations to anticipate the risks that are likely to occur in patients with limited lesion-specific data.

Guidelines

There are few guidelines focused on CHD, and most situations call for extrapolation of adult guidelines (**Table 2**). ICD implantation for secondary prevention due to irreversible causes remains a Class I indication in multiple guidelines, carrying the strongest level of evidence among recommendations in this group.[12,24] Most of the remaining recommendations are either supported by retrospective studies and case reports or are based on expert opinion.

Therapeutic Options and Surgical Techniques

Surgery, interventional catheterization, or cardiac ablation can modify sudden death substrate by addressing or eliminating ventricular pre-excitation, structural lesions, and coronary lesions. Medications are commonly used in the setting of

Table 1
Risk for all-cause mortality or ventricular tachycardia in tetralogy of Fallot

Factors	Odds Ratio	95% CI
Age (per year)[a,b]	1.04	1.03–1.05
Age at corrective surgery (per year)[a,b]	1.04	1.02–1.05
Prior palliative shunt[a,b]	2.80	1.83–4.28
Ventriculotomy[b]	2.18	1.26–3.78
Number of thoracotomies[a,b]	1.57	1.16–2.11
QRS duration (per ms)[a,b]	1.03	1.01–1.05
History of SVT/AF	1.94	1.09–3.46
RVEF (per 1% decrease), MRI	1.07	1.03–1.11
RV dysfunction at least moderate, echo[a,b]	2.04	1.32–3.16
RVESV (per 1 mL/m^2), MRI,[b]	1.02	1.01–1.03
LVEF (per 1% decrease), echo or MRI[b]	1.06	1.04–1.08

Abbreviations: AF, atrial fibrillation; echo, echocardiography; EF, ejection fraction; ESV, end-systolic volume; LV, left ventricle; MRI, magnetic resonance imaging; ms, millisecond; RV, right ventricle, SVT, supraventricular tachycardia.
   [a] Additional annotations mark factors that were also associated with VT.
   [b] Cardiac death and VT in separate analyses.
   Adapted from Possner and colleagues[23] Risk factors that did not meet statistical significance were removed from this summary table.

Table 2
A summary of the guidelines and expert consensus statements relevant to sudden death in congenital heart disease from 2012 to 2022

Year	Title	Notes
2021	The Pediatric and Congenital Electrophysiology Society (PACES) expert consensus statement on the indications and management of cardiovascular implantable electronic devices (CIED) in pediatric patients[12]	Extensive discussion of indications for CIED management in patients with congenital heart disease (CHD).
2019	American Heart Association/American College of Cardiology/Heart Rhythm Society (AHA/ACC/HRS) focused update of the 2014 AHA/ACC/HRS guideline for the management of patients with atrial fibrillation[57]	Does not address patients with CHD, but establishes basic principles of management that can be useful in this population.
2017	AHA/ACC/HRS guideline for management of patients with ventricular arrhythmias and the prevention of sudden cardiac death[58]	Contains a section specific to adult CHD and provides an overview of fundamental principles of medical and interventional management.
2017	ACC/AHA/HRS guideline for the evaluation and management of patients with syncope[59]	Contains specific sections on pediatric syncope and adult congenital heart disease.
2015	ACC/AHA/HRS guideline for the management of adult patients with supraventricular tachycardia[60]	Contains specific sections on pediatric arrhythmia and adult CHD.
2015	European Society of Cardiology (ESC) guidelines for the management of patients with ventricular arrhythmias and the prevention of sudden cardiac death[61]	Contains sections on pediatric arrhythmias and congenital heart disease. Complementary to the 2017 AHA/ACC/HRS guidelines.
2015	Eligibility and disqualification recommendations for competitive athletes with cardiovascular abnormalities	See both the preamble and general considerations,[62] as well as Task Force 4: CHD.[63]
2014	PACES/HRS expert consensus statement on the recognition and management of arrhythmias in adult congenital heart disease[64]	Focused on the needs of adults with CHD with recommendations on evaluation and therapy.
2012	American College of Cardiology Foundation/American Heart Association/Heart Rhythm Society (ACCF/AHA/HRS) focused update incorporated into the ACCF/AHA/HRS 2008 guidelines for device-based therapy of cardiac rhythm abnormalities[65]	Detailed discussion of indications for pacemakers and defibrillators.

arrhythmia risk, although data on quantitative risk reduction in CHD are scarce. For patients in whom treatment is already maximized or therapies to alter substrate are unavailable, reduction of sudden death risk may necessitate implantation of an ICD.

Catheter ablation of ventricular tachycardia (VT) or ventricular fibrillation (VF) is an important therapy to potentially reduce a patient's SCD risk.[25] However, there are scant data to daw conclusions about the effectiveness of ablation for most types of CHD, primarily due to the heterogeneity of anatomic substrates and successful ablation does not necessarily imply permanent elimination of sudden death risk. As mentioned previously, the most well-studied CHD lesion is ToF. Guidelines and extrapolations based on these studies may not be as useful when applied to single ventricle lesions or other types of CHD.

Historically, the correlation between VT/VF and SCD led to the practice of risk-stratifying patients by performing ventricular stimulation studies in the electrophysiology (EP) laboratory. However, subsequent multi-center studies showed that patients without clinical VT had a much lower positive predictive value from ventricular stimulation studies than patients with clinical VT. The Bayesian strategy is to use ventricular stimulation primarily in patients who fall in an intermediate risk category. Results of the study then inform posterior classification into lower or higher risk clinical categories.[25] Moreover, evaluation of risk factors has changed over time as the ToF population continues to survive into late adulthood. A national registry study in France found that in patients with certain risk characteristics, slower VT was more consistently associated with SCD. Elimination of these ventricular arrhythmias may avoid the need for ICD implantation in certain patients, but case-by-case judgment remains imperative.[26]

The substrate for VT in ToF primarily revolves around up to 4 anatomic isthmuses defined by areas of scar or suture lines created during surgical repair. These have been previously well-defined by Zeppenfeld and colleagues and include the area between the tricuspid valve and the right ventricular outflow tract (RVOT) patch, the area between the pulmonary valve and the RVOT patch, the area between the pulmonary valve and the ventricular septal defect (VSD) patch, and the area between the VSD patch and the tricuspid valve.[25,27–29] Not all of these isthmuses are present in every patient with ToF, and some are era-dependent due to changes in surgical technique.[25,29] During an EP study and ablation procedure, these isthmuses are mapped using multi-polar electrodes, and conduction velocities through these areas are calculated. The isthmuses with conduction velocities less than 0.5 m/s are targeted for ablation, and linear RF lesions are made between areas of unexcitable tissue (eg, scar, patch, or valve).[28]

Another important consideration for patients with ToF is how to manage ventricular tachycardia (VT) risk in the context of pulmonary valve replacement (PVR). Even though PVR can improve right ventricle (RV) hemodynamics, SCD from VT/VF remains a risk for these patients.[30] Complicating matters, the type of valve replacement may effectively render important regions of the RV later inaccessible for catheter ablation. Recent investigations have tried pre-emptively performing pre-PVR EP studies in patients undergoing transcatheter valve replacement.[30] However, this may uncover ventricular arrhythmias that are not clinically significant, resulting in interventions that may not be necessary at that particular time. Intraoperative ablation has also been suggested, although without concomitant intraoperative (and perhaps post-operative) mapping, it is difficult to ascertain the efficacy of these lesions in preventing future SCD.[30]

ICDs can provide anti-tachycardia pacing as well as defibrillation to abort life-threatening arrhythmias in patients with CHD. Many CHD patients can receive standard devices with a subclavian pulse generator and a defibrillation coil anchored in the right ventricle endocardium. In the current era, standard ICD implantation in structurally normal hearts is often performed without defibrillation threshold (DFT) testing and data support that choice.[31] However, few data are available on implanting ICDs without DFTs in CHD patients. Some centers omit routine DFTs in CHD patients with normal situs, normal device configurations, and a subjectively low risk of defibrillation failure, but this is on the basis of case-by-case risk-benefit calculations, rather than on the basis of data in the congenital population.

The standard transvenous approach is often infeasible for patients with CHD (**Fig. 3**A). Infants and small children have relatively narrow veins due to their small stature and are therefore at relatively high risk for venous obstruction over time. While adults and older children may be appropriately sized for a transvenous ICD, venous and intracardiac anomalies can prohibit this approach. Even a simple variation such as left superior vena cava with no bridging vein can add complexity to the procedure (see **Fig. 3**B). More complex heart diseases that include ventricular inversion or dextroposition can also affect the defibrillation vector (see **Fig. 3**D). CHD patients with residual intracardiac shunts are at higher risk for thromboembolic events.[32] Those with a mechanical or dysplastic tricuspid valve may not tolerate a lead through the valve, and lead placement in the setting of a cavopulmonary anastomosis is extremely challenging. In general, patients who receive atypical implantation techniques should still undergo some type of DFT testing at the time of implant.

New Technologies and Opportunities

In addition to traditional transvenous devices, congenital electrophysiologists have developed experience at collaborating or placing epicardial ICDs (**Fig. 3**E, F) and subcutaneous ICDs (**Fig. 3**C). Pediatric patients show a comparable rate of appropriate and inappropriate ICD shocks with use of transvenous and subcutaneous ICD systems, suggesting similar device fidelity[33]; however, many patients with CHD have abnormal repolarization, making accurate sensing a challenge. Medtronic has developed an extravascular ICD system in which the ICD coil is tunneled sub-sternally.[34] However, this device has not yet been rigorously reported in children or patients with CHD.

Future directions for ICD implantation include minimally invasive epicardial lead implantation.[35] This has potential applications for both infants

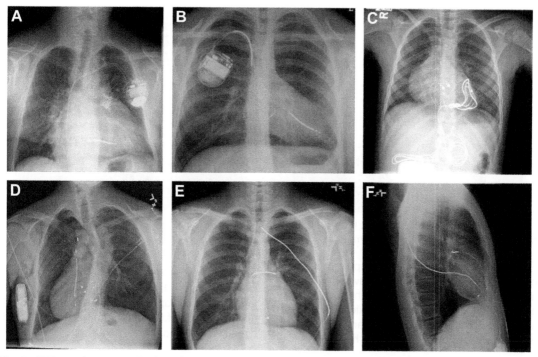

Fig. 3. CHD requires customized implantation strategies.(*A*). Traditional left-sided transvenous dual- chamber implantable cardioverter-defibrillator (ICD) system. (*B*) CHD patient with no bridging vein; a dual coil was used to provide adequate defibrillation vector. (*C*) Epicardial ICD patch. (*D*) Subcutaneous ICD for a patient with dextrocardia. (*E*) Epicardial and subcutaneous ICD coils placed to improve defibrillation vector. (*F*) Lateral view of the coils in E.

and small children as well as adults with CHD who have had previous sternotomies and have developed intrathoracic adhesions that can increase the morbidity and mortality of a redo sternotomy.[36,37]

Controversies and Complications

ICD risks generally fall into 2 broad categories: short-term risks associated with implantation, and long-term risks of the lead/device system itself (**Fig. 4**). Acute procedural risks of the transvenous approach include bleeding from the pocket or the venous access site, vascular injury to the veins or heart, and pneumothorax or hemothorax from vascular access and perforation that can lead to pericardial effusion, tamponade, or death. Subacute procedural risks include pocket infection or wound infection, and risk of erosion of the device.[38,39] Epicardial ICD implantation has additional procedural risks related to open chest surgery and pericardiotomy.

Overall, the need for ICD revision is higher in the CHD and pediatric populations.[40,41] Chronic risks of transvenous leads include venous stenosis and eventual lead failure. Transvenous lead extraction is a complex procedure associated with significant morbidity and mortality.[42,43] When no longer functional, epicardial leads are generally abandoned due to the high risk of trying to remove leads that are scarred down to the epicardium.[44] However, newer data have shown that there are long-term risks of coronary compression due to strangulation that can occur from scarring of epicardial leads over time.[44] The long-term risks of subcutaneous ICDs are still being defined in CHD.

The rate of ICD shock failure has been low in the adult population. Pediatric data show similar efficacy for first shock success as is seen in the adult population.[45] Software algorithms have also improved, with a goal of minimizing the risk of energy delivery for rhythms where shocks are ineffective.[46] Patients with CHD have a higher rate of inappropriate shocks than children with structurally normal hearts.[47,48] This is likely due to a combination of atrial arrhythmias and oversensing from abnormal repolarization.[45,46,48,49] Inappropriate shocks can result in serious psychological conditions such as anxiety and depression, and can significantly impact a patient's quality of life.[50] Several review articles are available with practical programming tips to reduce inappropriate shocks.[46,51,52]

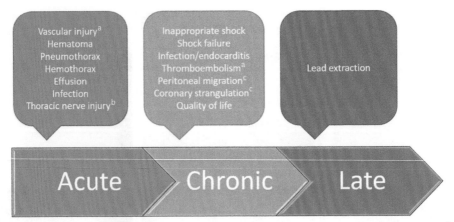

Fig. 4. Timeline of ICD complications. ICD risks and complications over time. [a] In transvenous systems; [b] In subcutaneous systems; [c] In epicardial systems.

ICDs are typically lifelong therapies and many patients feel constrained by the device.[53] Devices may visibly protrude, even through clothing, and all procedures leave a scar.[54] Anxiety and stress are elevated in children with ICDs and a therapeutic relationship with a counselor is helpful.[55,56]

SUMMARY

Assessment of sudden death risk should be a lifelong component of high-quality care in congenital heart disease. The 6 major risk factors for sudden death in CHD are underlying anatomy, symptoms, systemic ventricular function, atrial arrhythmias, ventricular arrhythmias, and pulmonary hypertension. The last 20 years have seen substantial advances in ablation and ICD care, but new technologies are in the pipeline just in time for an expanding population of CHD patients to receive optimal care.

CLINICS CARE POINTS

- Assessment of sudden death risk should be a lifelong component of high-quality care in CHD.
- The 6 major risk factors for sudden death in CHD are underlying anatomy, symptoms, systemic ventricular function, atrial arrhythmias, ventricular arrhythmias, and pulmonary hypertension.
- Assessing these 6 major risk factors requires substantial expertise in CHD and is optimally performed in a collaborative CHD environment.
- New technologies are in the pipeline just in time for an expanding population of CHD patients to receive optimal care.

FUNDING

Dr R. Kumthekar has received NIH, United States funding for development of novel devices for pediatric lead implantation. None of these devices are directly discussed in this manuscript.

DISCLOSURE

Dr R. Kumthekar has an ownership interest in PeriCor. No PeriCor device is directly discussed in this manuscript. No other disclosures to report.

REFERENCES

1. Pillutla P, Shetty KD, Foster E. Mortality associated with adult congenital heart disease: trends in the US population from 1979 to 2005. Am Heart J 2009;158(5):874–9.
2. Khairy P, Silka MJ, Moore JP, et al. Sudden cardiac death in congenital heart disease. Eur Heart J 2022;43(22):2103–15.
3. Bouchardy J, Therrien J, Pilote L, et al. Atrial arrhythmias in adults with congenital heart disease. Circulation 2009;120(17):1679–86.
4. Gallego P, Gonzalez AE, Sanchez-Recalde A, et al. Incidence and predictors of sudden cardiac arrest in adults with congenital heart defects repaired before adult life. Am J Cardiol 2012; 110(1):109–17.
5. Koyak Z, Harris L, de Groot JR, et al. Sudden cardiac death in adult congenital heart disease. Circulation 2012;126(16):1944–54.
6. Moore B, Yu C, Kotchetkova I, et al. Incidence and clinical characteristics of sudden cardiac death in adult congenital heart disease. Int J Cardiol 2018; 254:101–6.
7. Silka MJ, Hardy BG, Menashe VD, et al. A population-based prospective evaluation of risk of sudden cardiac death after operation for common

congenital heart defects. J Am Coll Cardiol 1998; 32(1):245–51.

8. Cobb LA, Fahrenbruch CE, Olsufka M, et al. Changing incidence of out-of-hospital ventricular fibrillation, 1980-2000. JAMA 2002;288(23):3008–13.

9. Oechslin EN, Harrison DA, Connelly MS, et al. Mode of death in adults with congenital heart disease. Am J Cardiol 2000;86(10):1111–6.

10. Rychik J, Atz AM, Celermajer DS, et al. Evaluation and Management of the Child and Adult With Fontan Circulation: A Scientific Statement From the American Heart Association. Circulation 2019;140(6):e234–84.

11. Aboulhosn JA, Lluri G, Gurvitz MZ, et al. Left and right ventricular diastolic function in adults with surgically repaired tetralogy of Fallot: a multi-institutional study. Can J Cardiol 2013;29(7):866–72.

12. Writing Committee M, Silka MJ, Silva JNA, et al. 2021 PACES expert consensus statement on the indications and management of cardiovascular implantable electronic devices in pediatric patients. Heart Rhythm 2021;18(11):1888–924.

13. Huntgeburth M, Hohmann C, Ewert P, et al. Implantable loop recorder for monitoring patients with congenital heart disease. Cardiovasc Diagn Ther 2021;11(6):1334–43.

14. Sakhi R, Kauling RM, Theuns DA, et al. Early detection of ventricular arrhythmias in adults with congenital heart disease using an insertable cardiac monitor (EDVA-CHD study). Int J Cardiol 2020;305:63–9.

15. Dodeja AK, Thomas C, Daniels CJ, et al. Detection of arrhythmias in adult congenital heart disease patients with LINQ(TM) implantable loop recorder. Congenit Heart Dis 2019;14(5):745–51.

16. Bezzerides VJ, Walsh A, Martuscello M, et al. The real-world utility of the LINQ implantable loop recorder in pediatric and adult congenital heart patients. JACC Clin Electrophysiol 2019;5(2):245–51.

17. Tsai SF, Chan DP, Ro PS, et al. Rate of inducible ventricular arrhythmia in adults with congenital heart disease. Am J Cardiol 2010;106(5):730–6.

18. Alexander ME, Walsh EP, Saul JP, et al. Value of programmed ventricular stimulation in patients with congenital heart disease. J Cardiovasc Electrophysiol 1999;10(8):1033–44.

19. Czosek RJ, Anderson J, Khoury PR, et al. Utility of ambulatory monitoring in patients with congenital heart disease. Am J Cardiol 2013;111(5):723–30.

20. Poh C, Hornung T, Celermajer DS, et al. Modes of late mortality in patients with a Fontan circulation. Heart 2020;106(18):1427–31.

21. Drakopoulou M, Nashat H, Kempny A, et al. Arrhythmias in adult patients with congenital heart disease and pulmonary arterial hypertension. Heart 2018; 104(23):1963–9.

22. Ruopp NF, Cockrill BA. Diagnosis and treatment of pulmonary arterial hypertension: a review. JAMA 2022;327(14):1379–91.

23. Possner M, Tseng SY, Alahdab F, et al. Risk factors for mortality and ventricular tachycardia in patients with repaired tetralogy of Fallot: a systematic review and meta-analysis. Can J Cardiol 2020;36(11): 1815–25.

24. Tracy CM, Epstein AE, Darbar D, et al. 2012 ACCF/AHA/HRS focused update of the 2008 guidelines for device-based therapy of cardiac rhythm abnormalities: a report of the American college of cardiology foundation/American heart association task force on practice guidelines. Heart Rhythm 2012;9(10): 1737–53.

25. Cohen MI, Khairy P, Zeppenfeld K, et al. Preventing arrhythmic death in patients with tetralogy of Fallot: JACC review topic of the week. J Am Coll Cardiol 2021;77(6):761–71.

26. Laredo M, Duthoit G, Sacher F, et al. Rapid ventricular tachycardia in patients with tetralogy of Fallot and implantable cardioverter-defibrillator: insights from the DAI-T4F nationwide registry. Heart Rhythm 2023;20(2):252–60.

27. Zeppenfeld K, Schalij MJ, Bartelings MM, et al. Catheter ablation of ventricular tachycardia after repair of congenital heart disease: electroanatomic identification of the critical right ventricular isthmus. Circulation 2007;116(20):2241–52.

28. Wallet J, Kimura Y, Zeppenfeld K. Ventricular tachycardia ablation in adult congenital heart disease. Card Electrophysiol Clin 2022;14(4):709–27.

29. Kapel GF, Sacher F, Dekkers OM, et al. Arrhythmogenic anatomical isthmuses identified by electroanatomical mapping are the substrate for ventricular tachycardia in repaired Tetralogy of Fallot. Eur Heart J 2017;38(4):268–76.

30. Krieger EV, Zeppenfeld K, DeWitt ES, et al. Arrhythmias in repaired tetralogy of Fallot: a scientific statement from the American heart association. Circ Arrhythm Electrophysiol 2022;15(11):e000084.

31. Kannabhiran M, Mustafa U, Acharya M, et al. Routine DFT testing in patients undergoing ICD implantation does not improve mortality: A systematic review and meta-analysis. J Arrhythm 2018;34(6): 598–606.

32. Khairy P, Landzberg MJ, Gatzoulis MA, et al. Transvenous pacing leads and systemic thromboemboli in patients with intracardiac shunts: a multicenter study. Circulation 2006;113(20):2391–7.

33. von Alvensleben JC, Dechert B, Bradley DJ, et al. Subcutaneous implantable cardioverter-defibrillators in pediatrics and congenital heart disease: a pediatric and congenital electrophysiology society multicenter review. JACC (J Am Coll Cardiol): Clinical Electrophysiology 2020;6(14):1752–61.

34. Friedman P, Murgatroyd F, Boersma LVA, et al. Efficacy and safety of an extravascular implantable cardioverter-defibrillator. N Engl J Med 2022;387(14): 1292–302.

35. Clark BC, Davis TD, El-Sayed Ahmed MM, et al. Minimally invasive percutaneous pericardial ICD placement in an infant piglet model: head-to-head comparison with an open surgical thoracotomy approach. Heart Rhythm 2016;13(5):1096–104.

36. Kumthekar RN, Sinha L, Opfermann JD, et al. Surgical pericardial adhesions do not preclude minimally invasive epicardial pacemaker lead placement in an infant porcine model. J Cardiovasc Electrophysiol 2020;31(11):2975–81.

37. Cannata A, Petrella D, Russo CF, et al. Postsurgical intrapericardial adhesions: mechanisms of formation and prevention. Ann Thorac Surg 2013;95(5):1818–26.

38. Stefanelli CB, Bradley DJ, Leroy S, et al. Implantable cardioverter defibrillator therapy for life-threatening arrhythmias in young patients. J Intervent Card Electrophysiol 2002;6(3):235–44.

39. Link MS, Hill SL, Cliff DL, et al. Comparison of frequency of complications of implantable cardioverter-defibrillators in children versus adults. Am J Cardiol 1999;83(2):263–6.

40. Dechert BE, Bradley DJ, Serwer GA, et al. Implantable cardioverter defibrillator outcomes in pediatric and congenital heart disease: time to system revision. Pacing Clin Electrophysiol 2016;39(7):703–8.

41. Baskar S, Bao H, Minges KE, et al. Characteristics and outcomes of pediatric patients who undergo placement of implantable cardioverter defibrillators: insights from the national cardiovascular data registry. Circ Arrhythm Electrophysiol 2018;11(9):e006542.

42. Gomes S, Cranney G, Bennett M, et al. Long-term outcomes following transvenous lead extraction. PACE - Pacing and Clinical Electrophysiology 2016;39(4):345–51.

43. Atallah J, Erickson CC, Cecchin F, et al. Multi-institutional study of implantable defibrillator lead performance in children and young adults results of the Pediatric Lead Extractability and Survival Evaluation (PLEASE) Study. Circulation 2013;127(24):2393–402.

44. Mah DY, Prakash A, Porras D, et al. Coronary artery compression from epicardial leads: more common than we think. Heart Rhythm 2018;15(10):1439–47.

45. Krause U, Müller MJ, Wilberg Y, et al. Transvenous and non-transvenous implantable cardioverter-defibrillators in children, adolescents, and adults with congenital heart disease: who is at risk for appropriate and inappropriate shocks? Europace 2019;21(1):106–13.

46. Garnreiter JM, Pilcher TA, Etheridge SP, et al. Inappropriate ICD shocks in pediatrics and congenital heart disease patients: risk factors and programming strategies. Heart Rhythm 2015;12(5):937–42.

47. Khairy P, Harris L, Landzberg MJ, et al. Implantable cardioverter-defibrillators in tetralogy of Fallot. Circulation 2008;117(3):363–70.

48. Berul CI, Van Hare GF, Kertesz NJ, et al. Results of a multicenter retrospective implantable cardioverter-defibrillator registry of pediatric and congenital heart disease patients. J Am Coll Cardiol 2008;51(17):1685–91.

49. Alexander ME, Cecchin F, Walsh EP, et al. Implications of implantable cardioverter defibrillator therapy in congenital heart disease and pediatrics. J Cardiovasc Electrophysiol 2004;15(1):72–6.

50. Czosek RJ, Bonney WJ, Cassedy A, et al. Impact of cardiac devices on the quality of life in pediatric patients. Circ Arrhythm Electrophysiol 2012;5(6):1064–72.

51. Khairy P, Mansour F. Implantable cardioverter-defibrillators in congenital heart disease: 10 programming tips. Heart Rhythm 2011;8(3):480–3.

52. Mansour F, Khairy P. Programming ICDs in the modern era beyond out-of-the box settings. Pacing Clin Electrophysiol 2011;34(4):506–20.

53. Mellion K, Uzark K, Cassedy A, et al. Health-related quality of life outcomes in children and adolescents with congenital heart disease. J Pediatr 2014;164(4):781–788 e1.

54. Durani P, McGrouther DA, Ferguson MW. The Patient Scar Assessment Questionnaire: a reliable and valid patient-reported outcomes measure for linear scars. Plast Reconstr Surg 2009;123(5):1481–9.

55. Sears SF, Hazelton AG, St Amant J, et al. Quality of life in pediatric patients with implantable cardioverter defibrillators. Am J Cardiol 2011;107(7):1023–7.

56. Webster G, Panek KA, Labella M, et al. Psychiatric functioning and quality of life in young patients with cardiac rhythm devices. Pediatrics 2014;133(4):e964–72.

57. Writing Group M, Wann LS, Calkins H, et al. 2019 AHA/ACC/HRS focused update of the 2014 AHA/ACC/HRS guideline for the management of patients with atrial fibrillation: a report of the American college of cardiology/American heart association task force on clinical practice guidelines and the heart rhythm society. Heart Rhythm 2019;16(8):e66–93.

58. Al-Khatib SM, Stevenson WG, Ackerman MJ, et al. 2017 AHA/ACC/HRS guideline for management of patients with ventricular arrhythmias and the prevention of sudden cardiac death: a report of the American college of cardiology/American heart association task force on clinical practice guidelines and the heart rhythm society. Heart Rhythm 2018;15(10):e73–189.

59. Shen WK, Shen WK, Sheldon RS, et al. 2017 ACC/AHA/HRS guideline for the evaluation and management of patients with syncope: a report of the American college of cardiology/American heart association task force on clinical practice guidelines, and the heart rhythm society. Heart Rhythm 2017;14(8):e155–217.

60. Page RL, Joglar JA, Caldwell MA, et al. 2015 ACC/AHA/HRS guideline for the management of adult patients with supraventricular tachycardia: a report of the American college of cardiology/American heart association task force on clinical practice guidelines and the heart rhythm society. J Am Coll Cardiol 2016;67(13):e27–115.

61. Priori SG, Blomström-Lundqvist C, Mazzanti A, et al. 2015 ESC guidelines for the management of patients with ventricular arrhythmias and the prevention of sudden cardiac death: the task force for the management of patients with ventricular arrhythmias and the prevention of sudden cardiac death of the European society of cardiology (ESC). Endorsed by: association for European paediatric and congenital cardiology (AEPC). Eur Heart J 2015;36(41):2793–867.

62. Maron BJ, Zipes DP, Kovacs RJ, et al. Eligibility and disqualification recommendations for competitive athletes with cardiovascular abnormalities: preamble, principles, and general considerations: a scientific statement from the American heart association and American college of cardiology. J Am Coll Cardiol 2015;66(21):2343–9.

63. Van Hare GF, Ackerman MJ, Evangelista JAK, et al. Eligibility and disqualification recommendations for competitive athletes with cardiovascular abnormalities: task force 4: congenital heart disease: a scientific statement from the American heart association and American college of cardiology. J Am Coll Cardiol 2015;132(22):e281–91.

64. Khairy P, Van Hare GF, Balaji S, et al. PACES/HRS expert consensus statement on the recognition and management of arrhythmias in adult congenital heart disease: developed in partnership between the pediatric and congenital electrophysiology society (PACES) and the heart rhythm society (HRS). Endorsed by the governing bodies of PACES, HRS, the American college of cardiology (ACC), the American heart association (AHA), the European heart rhythm association (EHRA), the Canadian heart rhythm society (CHRS), and the international society for adult congenital heart disease (ISACHD). Can J Cardiol 2014;30(10):e1–63.

65. Epstein AE, DiMarco JP, Ellenbogen KA, et al. 2012 ACCF/AHA/HRS focused update incorporated into the ACCF/AHA/HRS 2008 guidelines for device-based therapy of cardiac rhythm abnormalities: a report of the American college of cardiology foundation/American heart association task force on practice guidelines and the heart rhythm society. J Am Coll Cardiol 2013;61(3):e6–75.

66. Verheugt CL, Uiterwaal CSPM, van der Velde ET, et al. Mortality in adult congenital heart disease. Eur Heart J 2010;31(10):1220–9.

67. Zomer AC, Vaartjes I, Uiterwaal CSPM, et al. Circumstances of death in adult congenital heart disease. Int J Cardiol 2012;154(2):168–72.

68. Engelings CC, Helm PC, Abdul-Khaliq H, et al. Cause of death in adults with congenital heart disease - an analysis of the German National Register for Congenital Heart Defects. Int J Cardiol 2016;211:31–6.

Emerging Technologies for the Smallest Patients

Bradley C. Clark, MD[a],*, Charles I. Berul, MD[b]

KEYWORDS

- Cardiac implantable electronic device • Pediatrics • Pacemaker
- Implantable cardioverter defibrillator • Implantable cardiac monitor • Atrioventricular block
- Pericardial access • Miniaturization

KEY POINTS

- Pediatric patients and those with repaired and unrepaired congenital heart disease often have limited options for method of device implantation given the risk of venous occlusion, lack of intra-cardiac access, and paucity of subcutaneous tissue available for device generators.
- Device technology, including pacemaker/ICD generators have gotten smaller and have been significantly improved since their inception, but many still remain sub-optimal for the pediatric and congenital heart disease population.
- The development and integration of leadless pacing technology has added an additional option for pediatric patients and those with congenital heart disease requiring pacemaker therapy though concerns remain regarding implant issues, long-term device management, and retrieval.
- Fetal high-grade atrioventricular block carries a high risk for hydrops fetalis and fetal demise. Medical and procedural options are still lacking, though the development of a fetal micropacemaker is promising in pre-clinical testing.
- Lead implantation through a minimally invasive pericardial port approach offers a non-transvenous closed-chest option though this has not yet been validated in human infants.

INTRODUCTION

In 1954, Dr. Clarence Walton Lillehei published a series of 45 patients with congenital heart disease (including tetralogy of Fallot, atrioventricular septal defect, and ventricular septal defects) that he repaired.[1] In this series, he reported that 6 of the patients developed post-operative complete atrioventricular block (AVB) with 100% mortality. This led to work with Dr. John Johnson, who in 1956 utilized the Grass Physiologic Stimulator in a canine model to successfully pace the right ventricle using myocardial and skin electrodes.[2] The voltage required to pace the right ventricle was only 2 to 3 V but the pacemaker generator was the size of a microwave oven. Later in 1957, the same stimulator was used in a 2-year-old patient who had repair of a ventricular septal defect and developed post-operative complete AVB. With the use of the prototype pacemaker, this patient was able to survive to discharge. The team, working with Earl Bakken, who later founded Medtronic, Inc, developed a battery powered pacemaker that was first implanted in December 1957. This event was preceded by a major power outage in Minneapolis, Minnesota that led to a child's death due to a lack of emergency power backup in individual patient rooms. The development of an implantable cardioverter defibrillator (ICD) occurred more than 20 years later with the

[a] Division of Pediatric Cardiology, Department of Pediatrics, Masonic Children's Hospital, University of Minnesota Medical School, 2450 Riverside Avenue South, AO-405, Minneapolis, MN 55454, USA; [b] Division of Cardiology, Department of Pediatrics, Children's National Hospital, George Washington University School of Medicine, 111 Michigan Avenue, NW, Washington, DC 20010, USA
* Corresponding author.
E-mail address: bradleyclarkep@gmail.com
Twitter: @Bradley_C_Clark (B.C.C.)

Card Electrophysiol Clin 15 (2023) 505–513
https://doi.org/10.1016/j.ccep.2023.06.007
1877-9182/23/© 2023 Elsevier Inc. All rights reserved.

first implantation of an ICD in 1980, developed by Michel Mirowski and Morton Mower.[3]

CLINICAL RELEVANCE

The indications for the use of cardiac implantable electronic devices (CIED) in pediatric patients were recently updated as a Pediatric and Congenital Electrophysiology Society (PACES) Expert Consensus Statement.[4]

Pacemaker

There is a range of indications for pacemaker implantation in pediatric and adult congenital heart disease (ACHD) that includes sinus node dysfunction and high-grade AV block including congenital, acquired, and post-operative etiologies. Congenital AV block can be secondary to maternal systemic lupus erythematous (SLE) and other connective tissue disorders with anti-Ro/La antibodies, or can be associated with certain forms of congenital heart disease, but is often idiopathic. Congenital complete AVB can often lead to fetal demise and although fetal monitoring has improved earlier detection, there is currently no therapy that definitively prevents adverse outcomes.

Implantable Cardioverter Defibrillator

ICD implantation occurs in a variety of scenarios both in the form of primary and secondary prevention to prevent sudden cardiac death. Implantation of a secondary prevention ICD is performed in the setting of a patient who is the survivor of an aborted sudden cardiac arrest without a reversible etiology. Primary prevention ICD therapy in pediatric patients is usually indicated in patients with high-risk forms of inherited arrhythmia syndromes such as long QT syndrome, Brugada syndrome, and catecholaminergic polymorphic ventricular tachycardia, cardiomyopathy syndromes such as hypertrophic cardiomyopathy, dilated cardiomyopathy or arrhythmic cardiomyopathy or concerning cardiac family history. Not all patients with inherited arrhythmias or cardiomyopathies require ICD implantation, with patient selection and risk stratification remaining key clinical decision making issues.

Implantable Monitors

Compared to their adult counterparts, implantable cardiac monitors are performed less frequently in the pediatric population, but still have diagnostic utility in the right clinical scenarios. Infrequent symptoms such as palpitations or episodes of syncope or seizures of unclear etiology despite external monitoring may warrant the implant of a subcutaneous monitor with the potential of 2 to 4 years of monitoring with a single device. Additionally, pediatric patients with inherited arrhythmia or cardiomyopathy syndromes with symptomatic concerns but no clear device indication may benefit from an implantable monitor.

NATURE OF THE PROBLEM

Although the first description of an implanted pacemaker was in a pediatric patient with repaired congenital heart disease, children are now a tiny minority of patients receiving implantable devices. Small patients, especially those with challenging anatomic substrates, have more limited options for CIED implantation. Transvenous leads, while technically feasible in smaller children, may be less desirable due to the risk of vascular occlusion and subsequent inability to perform future implantations without requiring a relatively high-risk lead extraction procedure. The risk of venous occlusion is increased in the smallest patients and those that require multiple leads. Further, the lack of subcutaneous tissue in the pectoral region creates an elevated risk of skin complications and CIED infection. Vos and colleagues published a series of 7 patients under 10 kg that underwent implantation of a single-chamber transvenous pacemaker.[5] In this series, 2 of the patients developed subclavian vein occlusion and 2 required repair of their atrioventricular valve secondary to severe insufficiency. Two additional patients required intervention for imminent skin necrosis within 3 days of implant requiring revision and replacement of the generator pocket. However, it is more than simple age and size that portend venous obstruction in pediatric patients, as some older and larger children still can develop vascular issues following transvenous lead placement (**Fig. 1**).[6]

Additionally, patients with either repaired or unrepaired congenital heart disease (CHD) often have a lack of endocardial access or a single systemic ventricle where lead placement would lead to an unacceptable risk of thrombosis or endocarditis. Though there are occasional transvenous options in single ventricle patients, including the potential for transvenous atrial lead implantation in patients with Fontan circulation, most often in a lateral tunnel (**Fig. 2**). Patients with the presence of either congenital or residual atrial or ventricular septal defects are typically not considered candidates for transvenous devices due to an unacceptable risk of right-to-left shunt and resultant endocarditis, embolic phenomena or stroke.

Epicardial device implantation is an option for these patients but requires an invasive surgery

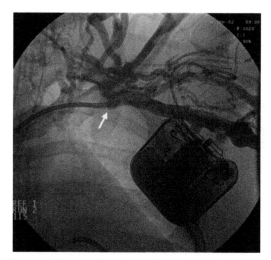

Fig. 1. Evidence of venous occlusion with collateralization in a patient with single-chamber transvenous ICD lead.[6] This lead is seen entering the left subclavian vein which is severely obstructed (*arrow*) as it traverses below the left clavicle. Collateral venous vessels form to compensate for the reduced flow through the subclavian vein and connect more proximally to drain into the superior vena cava.

through either a sternotomy/mini-sternotomy or thoracotomy with the generator most often placed in an abdominal sub-rectus pocket. These systems are often placed in smaller children and there is a substantial risk of lead fracture (**Fig. 3**) and device failure, especially during periods of rapid somatic growth. Subsequent procedures such as lead replacement or additional lead placement require re-sternotomy with the risk of bleeding and difficulty accessing functional myocardium

from scarring both on the epicardial surface and pericardium. Patients requiring implantation of an epicardial ICD create an even more challenging situation due to the difficulty of placement of the shocking coil in a non-transvenous location such as the pericardial (**Fig. 4**) or pleural space. There may be limited space and a challenge in creating an adequate shocking vector in order to produce life-saving electrical therapy. ICDs have much larger generators compared to pacemakers and there is a higher risk of skin complications, especially in the smallest patients.

The most challenging patient population regarding CIED implantation is low birth weight neonates. In cases of extreme prematurity (gestational age < 28 weeks), patient size is often inadequate for even the smallest pacemaker generator. When there is hemodynamically significant high-grade AVB, the placement of epicardial leads and a permanent pacemaker generator may not be feasible, particularly in the smallest neonates under 2 kg. In these cases, it may require either the placement of temporary epicardial pacemaker wires and an external temporary pacemaker generator or an externalized permanent pacing lead connected to standard implantable pulse generator until sufficient growth has occurred. Epicardial wires are at risk for fracture and elevated thresholds that are higher than can be provided by the temporary PM (usually maximum of 25 mA). Further, there is a risk of infection since the lead or wires and generator are externalized. If the temporary system is functional, the patient is monitored in an intensive care unit setting until adequate growth has been achieved to attempt an epicardial PM insertion.

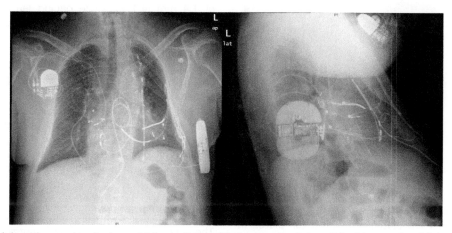

Fig. 2. Adult with complex single ventricle anatomy with Fontan circulation. Prior history of multiple epicardial devices with epicardial lead fracture. Patient underwent transvenous atrial lead implant from the right innominate vein into the Fontan circuit due to persistent brady-tachy syndrome, with right pectoral pacemaker generator; subsequently a subcutaneous ICD was implanted in the left chest due to the presence of ventricular arrhythmias.

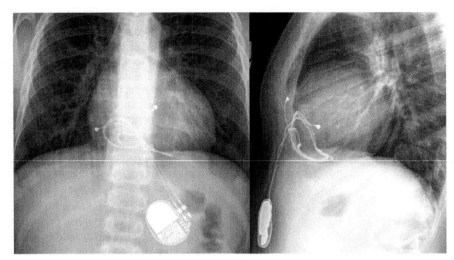

Fig. 3. Anteroposterior and lateral views demonstrating a visible conductor fracture on the atrial epicardial lead as it crosses diaphragm, likely secondary to patient somatic growth.

DISCUSSION
Miniaturization of both Leads and Generators

One of the most important trends since the first development of CIEDs has been the gradual decrease in the size of both pacemaker/ICD leads and generators. The current size range of pacemaker generators is 5 to 8 cc[7] which is a substantial

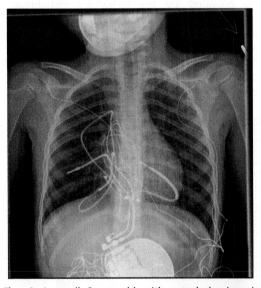

Fig. 4. A small 2-year-old with catecholaminergic polymorphic ventricular tachycardia who had suffered a ventricular fibrillation arrest underwent epicardial dual-chamber ICD placement, with a coil placed in the posterior pericardial space. The pace/sense lead is not utilized in this configuration, and is capped and put in the right pleural space. Epicardial sew-on pacing leads are seen on the right atrium and ventricle, and the ICD generator in mid-abdomen.

improvement from the pacemaker as large as a microwave. Defibrillator generators are much larger in size due to higher complexity and capacitors for shocking; the initial devices had displacement volumes ranging from 150 to 200 cc. Currently, the largest ICD generators (CRT devices with larger headers) range from 30 to 40 cc.[8]

Although pacing and defibrillation leads have become smaller in diameter, there remains a substantial risk of venous occlusion, especially in patients with small vasculature. Lead size also determines the size of sheath required for vascular access with larger sheaths increasing the potential for bleeding complications. An example of a current thinner pacemaker lead is the Medtronic SelectSecure 3830 which has an internal diameter of 1.4 mm (4.1 F), while pacing leads with an extendable/retractable screw are slightly larger, ranging from 5 to 6French. ICD leads are often larger due to the presence of shocking coils. For example, the Medtronic Sprint Quattro ICD lead has an internal diameter of 2.8 mm (8.6 F). Further miniaturization of these leads may not be feasible without sacrificing procedural success, lead stability, and risk of fracture. Recent attempts to produce a thinner defibrillator lead were fraught with a significantly higher rate of lead failure, which was exacerbated in the pediatric and congenital patients.[9]

Miniature Pacemaker

There has been a recent report of a surgical implant of an epicardial single-chamber PM (Louisville, KY, Norton Children's) using a prototype miniature pacemaker generator. The miniature pacemaker utilizes the Medtronic Micra leadless pacemaker as the generator and is connected to an epicardial lead. This procedure was performed in a premature neonate that was too small for the current pacemaker generators. Per report, the patient tolerated the procedure well without any complications related to implantation (personal communication). Since the initial implant, additional implants have been performed nationally (**Fig. 5**) with similar encouraging results.[10]

The potential to remarkably decrease the size of the pacemaker generator will likely increase the ability to perform minimally invasive or transvenous device implants in the smallest patients without the resultant increased risk of skin and infectious complications.

Fetal Micropacemaker

Fetal complete AV block and the risk of hydrops fetalis and fetal demise have led to the development of a micropacemaker with the potential capability to provide pacing to affected fetuses. The micropacemaker was designed with a lithium power cell and screw electrode with a flexible lead.[11,12] Initial in-vivo testing utilizing a conventional uterine cannula with an internal diameter of 3.3 mm was performed in a rabbit model.[11] Performance in a sheep model was performed with intermittent success though complications including pericardial effusion were encountered.[13] The team was able to perform successful implantation in the pericardial space in a pig model, though 5 out of 6 animals had either a lack of implantation

or were implanted and the system was non-functional.[14] While the success rate was low, the design of a novel micropacemaker has implications both for congenital complete AVB in the fetus but also for patients in the neonatal period and beyond. There continues to be an unmet need and enthusiasm for the potential development of a safe and reliable fetal pacemaker.

Leadless Pacing

With the development of leadless pacemakers such as the Medtronic Micra and the Abbott Aveir, there is the potential to avoid upper extremity venous access entirely and remove the risk of long-term damage to AV valves. In addition, there are advantages to avoid the need for a pre-pectoral or submuscular pocket.

Micra implantation has been documented in repaired CHD patients.[15] **Fig. 6** demonstrates Micra implantation in a 10-year-old patient with repaired tetralogy of Fallot/atrioventricular canal with post-operative complete AV block and a fractured epicardial lead.

Leadless pacing has been described in detail in chapter 3. Initial leadless pacemaker versions were only capable of single-chamber ventricular pacing. With newer versions such as the Micra AV and Aveir devices there is a potential for dual-chamber pacing. While not reported in a human subject, dual-chamber pacing with two leadless pacemakers (Abbott Aveir) and implant-to-implant communication has been evaluated in an

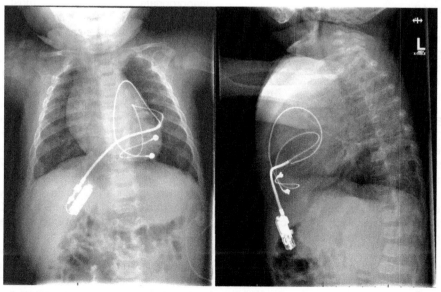

Fig. 5. Neonate, ex-32 week with prenatally diagnosed congenital complete AV block secondary to maternal anti-Ro/La antibodies. Patient was delivered pre-term for ventricular dysfunction and pericardial effusion and underwent prototype single-chamber epicardial PM with Micra generator ("Pediatric Implantable Pulse Generator") on the first day of life.

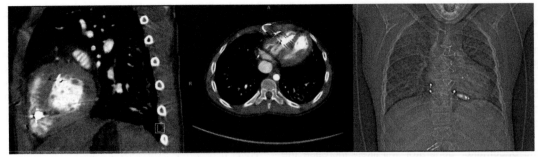

Fig. 6. 10 year old with repaired tetralogy of Fallot and complete atrioventricular canal who developed post-operative complete AV block. Initially underwent epicardial dual-chamber system but developed fracture of epicardial lead and underwent leadless Micra pacemaker implant to avoid additional surgical intervention.

ovine model.[16] Options for "dual-chamber" leadless pacing in addition to techniques combining transvenous and leadless devices may increase use of leadless pacing technology in pediatric patients.

Leadless Pacemakers in Clinical Trials

Aveir DR

The first in-human Aveir DR implant was performed in February 2022. This dual-chamber pacemaker is designed to provide synchronous, beat-by-beat pacing of the right atrium and right ventricle (RV). Its proprietary implant-to-implant (i2i) device technology is used for communication between 2 implanted leadless pacemakers for heart rate regulation.[17] Clinical trials are ongoing, and it is not currently available for commercial use.

EMPOWER LP

The EMPOWER LP by Boston Scientific is currently in clinical trials. This leadless pacemaker was designed to be paired with a subcutaneous defibrillator (Boston Scientific S-ICD) with unilateral communication between the devices to allow for anti-tachycardia pacing.[18]

The WiSE-CRT system

The WiSE-CRT system (EBR Systems, Sunnyvale, CA) is a leadless pacemaker designed to provide endocardial left ventricular (LV) pacing. This device consists of a receiver electrode (9.1 mm × 2.7 mm) that can be implanted via the retrograde or transeptal approach, a transmitter implanted in the intercostal space that can detect RV pacing and transmit ultrasound energy to the receiver electrode, and a battery.[19] The receiver electrode transforms the ultrasound energy into electrical energy which results in LV pacing. The safety and efficacy of this device are currently being investigated, and the device is approved for commercial use in Europe. Recently, the use of a WiSE-CRT system in combination with a leadless pacemaker to create a fully leadless CRT system was reported to demonstrate proof of concept.[20]

Subcutaneous Implantable Cardioverter Defibrillator

The subcutaneous ICD (S-ICD, Boston Scientific) was created to allow for the defibrillation of life-threatening arrhythmias without the need for intra-cardiac or surgical epicardial access. Initial models of the S-ICD did not have pacing capability and the first generation device had a large generator that would not be feasible for very small children. With the second generation device, the ICD generator size did decrease.

Von Alvensleben and colleagues published the largest cohort of pediatric and CHD patients (median 16.7 years) with the S-ICD.[21] Similar to published adult studies, there was a high rate of inappropriate shocks (15.6%), most frequently secondary to T-wave oversensing and sinus tachycardia. In this series, there was a low rate of both device erosion (0.8%) and infection (1.7%). Previously the youngest documented pediatric patient with an S-ICD was an 8 year old, 38 kg child with long QT syndrome who had an S-ICD implanted for secondary prevention.[22] A recent international series reported a total of 62 S-ICD implants in patients less than 18 years of age[23] and this series included a 3-year-old patient. Over a median follow-up period of 27 months, there was a 21% inappropriate shock incidence secondary to sinus tachycardia, supraventricular tachycardia, and T-wave oversensing. During the follow-up period, there were no reported deaths, lead fractures or device infections.

As the S-ICD device continues to evolve with the potential miniaturization of the lead and generator, it may be a desirable option for certain patients, especially those who do not require a substantial amount of pacing and have limited intra-cardiac access. A newer extravascular ICD with the potential for pause-prevention pacing and anti-tachycardia pacing, in addition to defibrillation, has been validated in adult patients,[24] but no pediatric implants have been reported.

Pericardial Devices/Access

Recent research has evaluated the potential of utilizing the pericardial space for lead implantation in pediatric patients. The main advantage of pericardial access would be the avoidance of a sternotomy/mini-sternotomy or thoracotomy for lead placement. Additionally, pericardial placement would avoid placing leads within the vascular space and endocardium and eliminate the risk of long-term vascular occlusion and valvar regurgitation. The initial description of pericardial lead placement was in an infant porcine model.[25] Minimally invasive pericardial access was obtained through a subxiphoid approach with thoracoscopic visualization. Needle access was obtained to the pericardial space under direct visualization followed by sheath access and ICD lead implantation in the space with a side-biting helix. This procedural technique was directly compared with an open epicardial surgical approach. There was no difference in lead measurements at implant and throughout the survival period and there was no significant change in defibrillation threshold testing at implant or at the end of the survival period between the 2 groups. A novel device was then developed that incorporated visualization and pericardial access and the procedure can be performed utilizing a single 10 mm incision in the subxiphoid area, which was demonstrated in an infant porcine model.[26] Developments have been made to minimize the size of the pacemaker generator utilizing the Micra leadless pacemaker with a leadlet which was successfully placed in the pericardial space in an infant porcine model.[27]

The subxiphoid approach and minimally invasive pericardial access for lead implantation have substantial potential advantages compared to the current approaches. This procedure can be performed by a pediatric electrophysiologist and would not require a congenital cardiovascular surgeon for device implantation. It creates an additional option for patients with prior sternotomy and CHD repair without requiring re-sternotomy and resultant risks. Although the presence of pericardial adhesions is a potential complicating factor for patients with prior cardiac surgery, the approach was validated and feasible in a pericardial adhesion model.[28]

Implantable Cardiac Monitor

Beyond the patients that require PM or ICD implantation, there are many additional individuals that require cardiac monitoring for concerning cardiac symptoms, inherited arrhythmia or cardiomyopathy syndromes not meeting indication for PM or ICD implant or concerning cardiac family history. For patients that require monitoring outside of the standard 30-day window for ambulatory cardiac monitor, the ICM gives an option for more prolonged monitoring. These small devices are placed in the subcutaneous area and currently can be performed either as an outpatient procedure or often with minimal sedation; the entire procedure typically takes 10 to 15 minutes to complete.

The first ICM (Reveal XT, Medtronic Inc) was introduced in 1990 and had a weight of 15 g, which was substantially larger than the 2nd generation (Reveal LINQ) which has a weight of 2.5 g[29] Currently, all major device companies, including Medtronic, Boston Scientific, St. Jude/Abbott, and Biotronik, have available ICMs that range in size from 1 to 6.5 cm.[30] The battery lives of these devices range from 2 to 4 years and allow continuous monitoring for patients at risk for either brady or tachyarrhythmias.

FUTURE DIRECTIONS

- Given the relative rarity of these conditions, the incidence of pediatric bradyarrhythmias and those conditions that create risk of sudden cardiac death are likely to remain stable over the coming years. Since medical therapies for many of these conditions are not available, pediatric and CHD patients will continue to have a need for CIED implantation.
- Technologies, including both leads and device generators, will trend toward miniaturization with improvement in battery longevity.
- With the elevated risk of epicardial CIED procedures, practitioners will likely choose alternative options, even for the youngest patients, including transvenous, pericardial, and leadless approaches.
- As the number of pediatric and CHD patients with leadless pacing increases, the comfort level for a pediatric electrophysiologist to implant and retrieve these devices will surely increase. Leadless pacemaker technology, especially related to the integration of atrial sensing, will further the suitability of these devices for pediatric patients.
- The continued development of rechargeable options for CIED generators may decrease the frequency of pacemaker generator replacement procedures.
- Treatment of congenital heart block and other fetal arrhythmia conditions is still challenging and despite heroic research efforts, a clinical fetal pacemaker has not yet been achieved.

SUMMARY

There is a large range and need for cardiac implantable electronic devices in pediatric patients including pacemakers, ICD and implantable cardiac monitors. Although both leads and generators have substantially decreased in size since inception, there remains a size discrepancy that can negatively impact patients. Specifically related to pacemakers and ICDs, the transvenous route is typically preferred for stability and procedural difficulty, but there are many limitations including patient size, septal defects and types of repaired and unrepaired congenital heart disease. Epicardial device implantations are often necessary but require a congenital surgeon and have multiple limitations including a higher risk of lead fracture and challenging re-interventions. While options including leadless pacing and pericardial lead implantation may be promising, they are currently not ready for primetime with regards to the pediatric and congenital populations. Pediatric providers will continue to require outside of the box thinking to care for our patients as emerging technologies become more available to pediatric electrophysiologists.

CLINICS CARE POINTS

- While there is no specific weight cutoff for transvenous device implantation in pediatric patients, the performance in children less than 10 kg may create an increased risk of venous occlusion, skin complications and atrioventricular valve regurgitation.
- Transvenous lead implantation should not be performed in a systemic atria or ventricle or in patients with atrial or ventricular septal defects.
- Epicardial cardiac devices require surgical implantation, sternotomy or thoracotomy and often have an elevated risk of bleeding or inadequate lead parameters secondary to re-sternotomy and pericardial adhesions.
- The smallest neonates require special attention due to a lack of adequate subcutaneous tissue for a device generator. These patients may require epicardial wire placement for temporary pacing to allow for adequate growth prior to epicardial lead and generator implant.
- The implantation of a loop recorder in pediatric patients has multiple indications including concerning symptoms and risk factors for AV block or sudden cardiac events. These devices are small in nature and the

procedure can typically be performed with minimal sedation.

- There are no current defined indications for leadless pacemaker implantation in the pediatric or congenital heart disease population though their use may increase with improvement in dual-chamber pacing capability. The decision to proceed with leadless pacemaker must include the discussion of all risks, benefits, and alternatives with the patient and family.
- Pericardial access is currently utilized for procedures such as epicardial ablation and may be a useful method for pediatric and congenital lead implantation.

DISCLOSURE

B.C. Clark and C.I. Berul have intellectual property and small business stake in PeriCor, LLC, which is the controlling company for a device that is referenced in this article. C.I. Berul has received research grants from Medtronic, Inc.

REFERENCES

1. Lillehei CW, Gott VL, Hodges PC Jr, et al. Transitor pacemaker for treatment of complete atrioventricular dissociation. J Am Med Assoc 1960;172:2006–10.
2. Gott VL. Critical role of physiologist John A. Johnson in the origins of Minnesota's billion dollar pacemaker industry. Ann Thorac Surg 2007;83(1):349–53.
3. Hauser RG. Development and Industrialization of the implantable cardioverter-defibrillator: a personal and historical perspective. Card Electrophysiol Clin 2009;1(1):117–27.
4. Shah MJ, Silka MJ, Silva JNA, et al. 2021 PACES Expert Consensus statement on the indications and management of cardiovascular implantable electronic devices in pediatric patients: developed in collaboration with and endorsed by the heart rhythm society (HRS), the American college of cardiology (ACC), the American heart association (AHA), and the association for European paediatric and congenital cardiology (AEPC) endorsed by the asia pacific heart rhythm society (APHRS), the Indian heart rhythm society (IHRS), and the Latin American heart rhythm society (LAHRS). JACC Clin Electrophysiol 2021;7(11):1437–72.
5. Vos LM, Kammeraad JAE, Freund MW, et al. Long-term outcome of transvenous pacemaker implantation in infants: a retrospective cohort study. Europace 2017;19(4):581–7.
6. Bar-Cohen Y, Berul CI, Alexander ME, et al. Age, size, and lead factors alone do not predict venous obstruction in children and young adults with

transvenous lead systems. J Cardiovasc Electrophysiol 2006;17(7):754–9.

7. Mallela VS, Ilankumaran V, Rao NS. Trends in cardiac pacemaker batteries. Indian Pacing Electrophysiol J 2004;4(4):201–12.

8. ICD technology. Int J Arrhythm 2011;12(4):10–5.

9. Atallah J, Erickson CC, Cecchin F, et al. Multi-institutional study of implantable defibrillator lead performance in children and young adults: results of the Pediatric Lead Extractability and Survival Evaluation (PLEASE) study. Circulation 2013;127(24): 2393–402.

10. Berul CI, Dasgupta S, LeGras MD, et al. Tiny pacemakers for tiny babies. Heart Rhythm 2023;20(5): 766–9.

11. Loeb GE, Zhou L, Zheng K, et al. Design and testing of a percutaneously implantable fetal pacemaker. Ann Biomed Eng 2013;41(1):17–27.

12. Zhou L, Vest AN, Peck RA, et al. Minimally invasive implantable fetal micropacemaker: mechanical testing and technical refinements. Med Biol Eng Comput 2016;54(12):1819–30.

13. Bar-Cohen Y, Loeb GE, Pruetz JD, et al. Preclinical testing and optimization of a novel fetal micropacemaker. Heart Rhythm 2015;12(7):1683–90.

14. Bar-Cohen Y, Silka MJ, Hill AC, et al. Minimally invasive implantation of a micropacemaker into the pericardial space. Circ Arrhythm Electrophysiol 2018; 11(7):e006307.

15. McGill M, Roukoz H, Jimenez E, et al. Leadless pacemaker placement in a pediatric tetralogy of Fallot patient with previous transcatheter valve replacement. J Electrocardiol 2019;56:52–4.

16. Cantillon DJ, Gambhir A, Banker R, et al. Wireless communication between paired leadless pacemakers for dual-chamber synchrony. Circ Arrhythm Electrophysiol 2022;15(7):e010909.

17. Aveir DR i2i Study. Available at: https://clinicaltrials. gov/show/NCT05252702. Accessed June 12, 2023.

18. Effectiveness of the EMPOWER™ Modular Pacing System and EMBLEM™ Subcutaneous ICD to Communicate Antitachycardia Pacing. Available at: https://clinicaltrials.gov/show/NCT04798768. Accessed June 12, 2023.

19. Singh JP, Abraham WT, Auricchio A, et al. Design and rationale for the stimulation of the left ventricular endocardium for cardiac resynchronization therapy in non-responders and previously untreatable patients (SOLVE-CRT) trial. Am Heart J 2019;217: 13–22.

20. Carabelli A, Jabeur M, Jacon P, et al. European experience with a first totally leadless cardiac resynchronization therapy pacemaker system. Europace 2021;23(5):740–7.

21. von Alvensleben JC, Dechert B, Bradley DJ, et al. Subcutaneous implantable cardioverter-defibrillators in pediatrics and congenital heart disease: a pediatric and congenital Electrophysiology society multicenter review. JACC Clin Electrophysiol 2020;6(14):1752–61.

22. Sarubbi B, Colonna D, Correra A, et al. Subcutaneous implantable cardioverter defibrillator in children and adolescents: results from the S-ICD "Monaldi care" registry. J Interv Card Electrophysiol 2022; 63(2):283–93.

23. Mori H, Sumitomo N, Tsutsui K, et al. Efficacy of SubcutAneous implantable cardioVErter-defibrillators in ≤18 year-old CHILDREN: SAVE-CHILDREN registry. Int J Cardiol 2023;371:204–10.

24. Friedman P, Murgatroyd F, Boersma LVA, et al. Efficacy and safety of an extravascular implantable cardioverter-defibrillator. N Engl J Med 2022;387(14): 1292–302.

25. Clark BC, Davis TD, El-Sayed Ahmed MM, et al. Minimally invasive percutaneous pericardial ICD placement in an infant piglet model: head-to-head comparison with an open surgical thoracotomy approach. Heart Rhythm 2016;13(5):1096–104.

26. Clark BC, Opfermann JD, Davis TD, et al. Single-incision percutaneous pericardial ICD lead placement in a piglet model. J Cardiovasc Electrophysiol 2017;28(9):1098–104.

27. Kumthekar RN, Opfermann JD, Mass P, et al. Percutaneous epicardial placement of a prototype miniature pacemaker under direct visualization: an infant porcine chronic survival study. Pacing Clin Electrophysiol 2020;43(1):93–9.

28. Kumthekar RN, Sinha L, Opfermann JD, et al. Surgical pericardial adhesions do not preclude minimally invasive epicardial pacemaker lead placement in an infant porcine model. J Cardiovasc Electrophysiol 2020;31(11):2975–81.

29. Bisignani A, De Bonis S, Mancuso L, et al. Implantable loop recorder in clinical practice. J Arrhythm 2019;35(1):25–32.

30. Trohman RG, Huang HD, Sharma PS. The miniaturization of cardiac implantable electronic devices: advances in diagnostic and therapeutic modalities. Micromachines 2019;10(10). https://doi.org/10. 3390/mi10100633.

Translation of Tools and Techniques from the Adult Electrophysiology World to Pediatric Cardiac Implantable Electronic Devices

Taylor S. Howard, MD[a],*, Jeffrey M. Vinocur, MD[b]

KEYWORDS

• Pediatric • Electrophysiology • Pacemaker • Implantable cardioverter defibrillator • CIED

KEY POINTS

- Detail current preoperative measures used in adults that could be applied to pediatric/congenital patients.
- Discuss the use of equipment and techniques designed for adults and opportunities to translate to pediatric/congenital patients.
- Explore pacemaker/implantable cardioverter defibrillator algorithms that have been used in adults but could be applied to pediatric/congenital patients.

INTRODUCTION

Self-contained, cardiac implantable electronic devices (CIEDs) were first used in humans beginning in 1958 when Ake Senning implanted the first permanent pacemaker in a 40-year-old patient.[1] Within 2 years, Larry Graves became the first child to have a pacemaker implanted after suffering complete atrioventricular (AV) block following cardiac surgery.[2,3] This device was implanted using a combined team of both pediatric and adult operators.[3] Since that time, the world of pediatric device therapy has coevolved with adult electrophysiology, now unavoidably, with adult-focused industry being the primary driver of CIED innovation. Given that pediatric CIED implants make up less than 1% of the 300,000 devices implanted each year in the United States alone,[4,5] there is less incentive for the development of pediatric-specific devices but indirect benefit accrues from advancements in technology (smaller devices, more physiologic pacing), implant techniques, and perioperative management. Pediatric and congenital electrophysiologists are caring for more complex young people than ever before and should remain alert to opportunities to innovate and translate novel techniques from the adult laboratory to the pediatric space.

Throughout the review of pediatric CIEDs presented in this edition of Clinics in Cardiac Electrophysiology, there are specific articles written on most types of devices. Our goal with this review is to look specifically at how the implant procedure and device programming can benefit from adult tools and techniques. We also discuss some common pediatric/congenital scenarios where typical adult-based tools have been adapted in unique ways, as well as to look forward to further collaborative opportunities.

[a] Department of Pediatrics, Division of Pediatric Cardiology, Baylor College of Medicine, Texas Children's Hospital, 6651 Main Street, E1920, Houston, TX 77030, USA; [b] Department of Pediatrics, Division of Pediatric Cardiology, Yale School of Medicine, 333 Cedar Street, New Haven, CT 06510, USA
* Corresponding author.
E-mail address: tshoward@bcm.edu

Card Electrophysiol Clin 15 (2023) 515–525
https://doi.org/10.1016/j.ccep.2023.06.004
1877-9182/23/© 2023 Elsevier Inc. All rights reserved.

IMPLANT PROCEDURE
Access

Obtaining safe and efficient vascular access is a key portion of the implant procedure for traditional CIEDs. In the earlier days of implantation, intrathoracic subclavian access was taught due to its relatively high success rates. This technique, however, came with a higher risk of pneumothorax and subclavian crush and therefore has given way to other means of access.[6–8] Because the subclavian vein crosses lateral to the first rib, it becomes extrathoracic, transitioning into the axillary vein (**Fig. 1**A). Within pediatrics, extrathoracic subclavian and axillary access have been advocated due to lower risk of complications[9] but may be challenging to implement consistently with the relatively low-CIED volumes encountered by many pediatric operators. Adult implanters have developed various techniques to assist the operator in gaining access with greater precision and safety.

For those who prefer fluoroscopy-guided venous access, a valuable technique is 35° caudal angulation on fluoroscopy (**Fig. 1**B, C). This technique highlights the anterior border of the lung and the first rib and allows for axillary access while avoiding potential intrathoracic puncture and thus pneumothorax.[10] The technique may be performed without venography but we have found that venography road map is additive to this technique.

Ultrasound access has also been shown to be successful, safe, and efficient in adult populations.[11–14] Authors describe the so-called out-of-plane technique or short axis and the in-plane technique or long axis (**Fig. 2**). These facilitate effective puncture by allowing for direct visualization of needle, vein, and adjacent structures. Although there is no firm evidence for a reduction in overall complications,[14] there is evidence for the reduction of fluoroscopy exposure.[15] Ultrasound can permit combined pectoral nerve block and axillary venipuncture[16] and preincisional vascular access[12] reducing radiation dose and eliminating the need for contrast administration. This technique has been found to be safe and effective in a pediatric and adult congenital heart disease (ACHD) population.[17]

Finally, cephalic vein cut down has been a popular alternative access used by adults.[18] This modality eliminates pneumothorax risk and has also been shown to have improved stability of leads.[19] The relatively small size of this vessel in pediatric patients may preclude its routine use but it can be considered selectively where venipuncture is difficult due to obesity or other factors.

Pacing Lead Implantation

Location of routine transvenous, right ventricular (RV) pacing leads has been a subject of debate for some time. Both adult and pediatric studies show high-pacing burden imposes risk for pacemaker-induced cardiomyopathy.[20–22] Thus, investigators have set out to discern if specific pacing sites protect against dyssynchrony and dysfunction. Although overall evidence is limited and mixed, RV septal pacing has emerged as potentially superior as compared with RV apical pacing.[21,23,24] In addition, it prevents cardiac perforation and helix-related reactive pericarditis, which can both be seen with any free-wall site, including the apex. Many pediatric implanters target the mid-RV septum but this is not easy to accomplish, with leads tending to end up in the anterior RV recess. Numerous tools and techniques have been developed for directing the lead toward the RV septum, and studies have detailed fluoroscopic techniques to ensure appropriate placement.

Septal lead placement is generally attempted using stylets or delivery sheaths/catheters. Classically, the "Mond Curve" stylet has been used to achieve routine access to the septum in stylet-driven leads with good success[25]; hand-shaped equivalents are commonly used but the success rate may vary. In addition, there are also deflectable stylets known as the Locator, available from Abbott (Abbott, Sylmar, CA, USA), which allow for a more tailored approach in the setting of challenging anatomy. Medtronic (Medtronic, Inc; Minneapolis, MN, USA), Boston Scientific (Boston Scientific, Natick, MA, USA), and Biotronik (Biotronik, Berlin, Germany), each have developed a series of precurved sheaths/catheters to facilitate access to various locations within the RV and the atria. One of the more popular leads in pediatrics is the Medtronic Select Secure 3830 lead (Medtronic, Inc; Minneapolis, MN, USA). This lead's 4.1-Fr diameter has facilitated its use in smaller patients and its recent approval for use in left bundle area pacing has also increased its use in adult electrophysiology (EP) (**Fig. 3**A). The 3830 lead is classically delivered by the Medtronic delivery catheters (**Fig. 3**B). Within this series, there are precurved options presenting numerous choices designed for locations including unusual atrial locations (see **Fig. 3**B). Among these, 4 have dual curvature similar to the Mond stylet to provide septal angulation (C315 His, C315 S4, C315 S5, and C315 S10). The C315 His is popular due to widespread use in conduction system pacing but its length (43 cm plus the hub) mandates the use of leads that are relatively long. The S4 and S5 models are shorter (30 cm plus the hub)

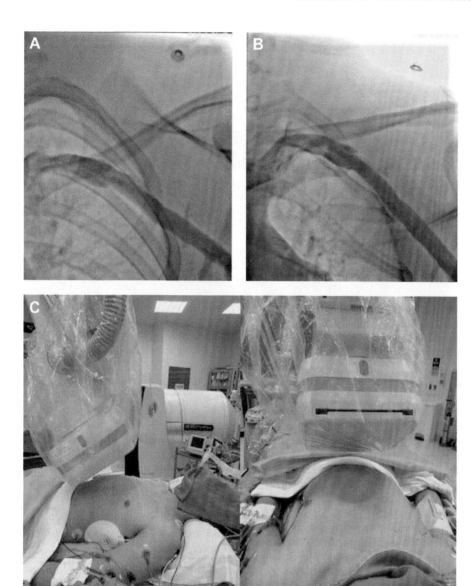

Fig. 1. (*A*) Axillary/subclavian venous anatomy in traditional frontal projection. The segment of vein to be accessed overlaps the lung field, and needle depth cannot be assessed radiographically. (*B*) Axillary/subclavian venous anatomy using caudal 35° tilt. The vein moves to the upper part of the screen and the lung to the lower part of the screen. Needle depth can be judged radiographically, and pneumothorax avoided. (*C*) Caudal angulation is easily accomplished and provides good exposure to the pectoral region for needle manipulation while fluoroscopy is used for guidance.

thus allowing the use of shorter leads with less slack to manage within the pocket. Although designed for atrial septal pacing, these work very well to achieve midventricular septal lead location in smaller patients. In fact, there has been one reported case of pediatric left bundle branch area pacing with this catheter.[26] Finally, there are also deflectable catheters available for additional flexibility (**Fig. 3**C).

Although these tools have proven extremely helpful in guiding lead placement, they do not guarantee septal position. Adult literature has established that many leads deemed midseptal by the implanter are not when cross-sectional imaging was used.[27] The intraventricular septum is a posterior structure and oblique in nature. The traditional criterion, lead pointing toward the spine in the left anterior oblique (LAO) view, turns out not to be a reliable predictor of septal lead placement.[27,28] Instead, confirming lead tip directed posteriorly in the left lateral view was superior in its ability to predict septal lead placement,[29,30] although lateral

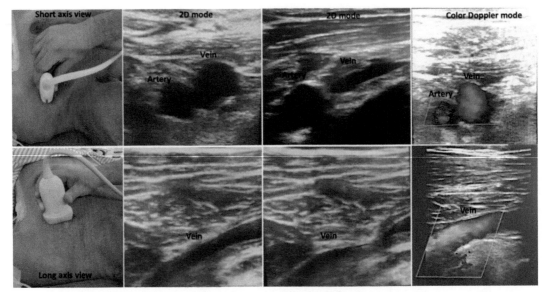

Fig. 2. Ultrasound imaging of axillary vein and artery. The axillary vein can be identified by its medial position, phasic (nonpulsatile) flow, and compressibility. Two different image planes can be acquired with probe either perpendicular or parallel to the vessel or needle. (*Adapted from* Tagliari et al, Heart Rhythm, 2013.[13])

fluoroscopy can be impractical depending on patient and laboratory setups. In these cases, a recent article from Squara and colleagues has suggested that an individualized LAO projection with 15° caudal angulation more accurately predicted a septal placement. In this technique, the implanter first finds the "individualized LAO angle by progressively aligning a posterior landmark (usually a guidewire spanning from superior vena cava [SVC] to inferior vena cava [IVC]) with an apical landmark (typically the RV lead or a pacing catheter). This aligns the eye to the lateral orientation of the septum. Then 15° caudal angulation is added, and the lead is placed toward the spine. The addition of caudal angulation allows the operator to identify the superior and inferior parts of

the septum. Using this technique, the team had excellent results.[31]

In practice, consistent, successful lead placement into the RV septum (or in left bundle branch area), improves with an understanding of patient-specific anatomy and various fluoroscopy techniques. When this knowledge is used in combination with modern stylets or sheaths, operators should be able to achieve the desired lead location.

Implantable Cardioverter Defibrillator Lead Implantation

Use of "coronary sinus" sheaths for additional support during RV lead placement is one valuable technique developed in the adult world (motivated

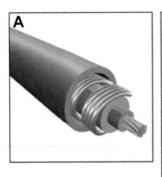 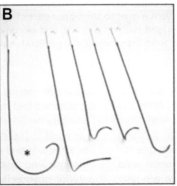 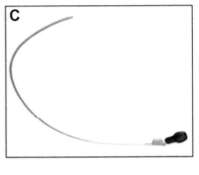

Fig. 3. (*A*) Select Secure 3830 lead has a coaxial construction without a stylet lumen. (*B*) Series of nondeflectable catheters used to deliver 3830 leads, asterisk indicates the C315 His catheter. (*C*) C304 deflectable catheter; a version with septal curve is also now available, not shown. (*Adapted from* Dandamudi et al, Heart Rhythm 2016.[60] All products from Medtronic [Medtronic, Inc.; Minneapolis, MN, USA].)

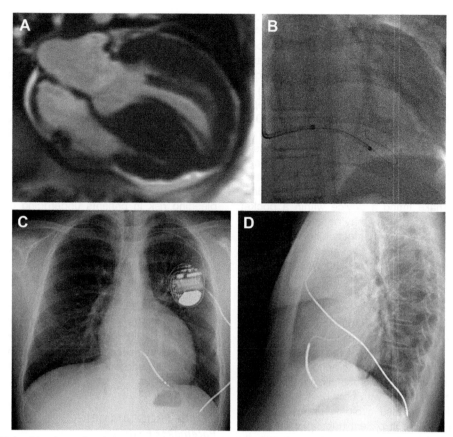

Fig. 4. ICD lead implantation in a patient with severe hypertrophic cardiomyopathy. (*A*) Cardiac MRI 4-chamber view shows near-obliteration of the RV cavity from the midventricular level. (*B*) The RV apex is accessed atraumatically using a coaxial system of Worley CS guide sheath, Worley "braided core," and soft guidewire; once the sheath is at the apex, a 9-Fr ICD lead is placed through it and fixated. (*C* and *D*) as the are an AP and Lateral of the same patient, i.e. different angles of view.

by right heart enlargement and tricuspid regurgitation seen secondarily in patients with heart failure). This can be used with pacing leads but is most useful for implantable cardioverter defibrillator (ICD) leads. Because the sheaths used for cardiac resynchronization therapy (CRT) implants are mostly 7-Fr inner diameter, ICD leads will typically require the "Worley" 9-Fr CS guide sheath (Merit Medical, South Jordan, UT), which comes with both a traditional dilator and a torqueable "inner core" that can be used to steer to a target location.

Besides the many patients with congenital right heart disease, this approach can also benefit children with severe hypertrophic cardiomyopathy and RV cavity distortion or obliteration. In these patients, manipulation of a relatively stiff ICD lead can be difficult, with associated risks (including perforation, proarrhythmia, and mechanical injury to the conduction system). A sheath-based approach, leading with a guidewire or soft catheter, can achieve an apical location gently and efficiently (**Fig. 4**).

Avoidance of Postimplantation Complications

One of the most dreaded complications following CIED implantation is infection. Despite modern antimicrobials, infection still largely requires device removal to clear the organism and thus is associated with increased health-care utilization and mortality.[32] Moreover, device-related infection is not necessarily a rare problem. A large Danish database publication consisting of 97,750 adult patients and 566,275 device-years revealed the lifetime risk of infection following implantation of CIEDs ranged from 1.6% to 3.4% depending on type of device implanted.[33] Predictably, ICDs and cardiac resynchronization thearpy + defibrillator (CRT-D) devices were at the highest risk. There also is a suggestion that infectious complications are more prevalent within the pediatric population.[34] This has resulted in institution-specific antibiotic prophylaxis protocols that are often more intense than suggested by the adult-based guidelines.[35] One tool that has promise to assist with protection against device infections is an antibiotic-impregnated covering. The WRAP-IT study randomized adult patients undergoing CIED implantation to the use of an absorbable antibiotic-eluting envelope. The trial showed a reduction in major device infections leading to removal or revision at 12 months. More in-depth analysis showed that patients undergoing ICD or CRT-D recipients were the only subgroup to have a significant reduction in major infections.[36] This study was reanalyzed at 21 months and continued to show a significant reduction in major infections.[37] Although the envelopes are expensive and make fitting a device within a pocket more cumbersome, they may be of benefit in patients at higher risk of infection, or where the adverse consequences of an infection would be greater. Further studies in pediatric/ACHD populations are warranted moving forward.

Pocket bleeding is an important predictor of device-related infection, and a troublesome complication in general. Pediatric and ACHD patients are becoming increasingly complex, with many on systemic anticoagulation. Adult implanters have had to deal with anticoagulated patients in high volumes and useful literature exist in guiding the implanter with how best to keep patients safe while also avoiding undue bleeding risk. Within the adult patient population, the data suggests that uninterrupted warfarin dramatically reduces bleeding risk (3.5% vs 16%) compared with using a heparin bridge strategy.[38] Therefore, most routine device procedures can proceed if the international normalized ratios (INRs) are not supratherapeutic.[38] Direct oral anticoagulants have become popular alternatives to warfarin for many indications in patients with ACHD, and in children, rivaroxaban is now US Food and Drug Administration (FDA) approved for deep vein thrombosis and for Fontan prophylaxis.[39] In the BRUISE CONTROL-2 trial, patients with moderate-to-high risk of arterial thromboembolic events had no higher risk of pocket bleeding with continued direct oral anticoagulants (DOAC) therapy in comparison with suspending DOACs surrounding this procedure.[40] Antiplatelet therapy, especially aspirin, is common in patients with congenital heart disease and does increase bleeding risk in patients undergoing device implantation.[41] This is especially true if used in conjunction with oral anticoagulation where it has been shown to be an independent risk factor in pocket bleeding.[42] There is not robust evidence on how to manage these medications at time of implant; individual risk/benefit analysis may favor holding aspirin for many of the indications in patients with ACHD (such as prevention of homograft conduit dysfunction). **Table 1** shows a brief outline of current evidence-based adult practices surrounding periprocedural management of anticoagulation.

DEVICE PROGRAMMING
Pacemaker Features

Progress in device programming has advanced rapidly, and current devices are nimbler and more physiologic than earlier generation devices. Device innovations are largely developed by manufacturers and, as such, typically target problems

Table 1
Adult evidence-based practice surrounding periprocedural anticoagulation

Anticoagulation/ Antithrombotic Management Medication	Lower Risk of Thrombosis	Higher Risk of Thrombosis	Evidence
Warfarin	Continue med, INR <3	Continue med, INR <3.5	Birnie et al,[38] 2013
DOAC	No definite recommendation but suspending therapy (without bridging) is reasonable in most cases with restart 48–72 h after procedure	Continue med	Birnie et al,[40] 2018; Du et al,[59] 2014
Antiplatelet	No definite recommendation but suspending therapy (without bridging) is reasonable in most cases with restart 48–72 h after procedure[a]	No definite recommendation, caution advised if concomitant dual agent platelet inhibitor or concomitant use with DOAC or warfarin	Notaristefano et al,[41] 2020; Essebag et al,[42] 2019

[a] Aspirin must be stopped 7 d before procedure for complete clinical effect.

common in adults. Nonetheless, given access to these programming features, the pediatric and ACHD implanter is benefited by understanding the programming basics and literature behind these various modalities. Perhaps, the last major advance in dual-chamber pacing was to limit unnecessary ventricular pacing. First developed as "managed ventricular pacing" or "MVP" (Medtronic, Inc.; Minneapolis, MN, USA),[43] most major device manufacturers offer similar algorithms, including ventricular intrinsic preference (Abbott, Sylmar, CA, USA), Vp suppression (Biotronik, Berlin, Germany), and AV Search + Rhythm IQ (Boston Scientific, Natick, MA, USA). Although the development of this modality predated the DAVID and MOST trials, it was the discovery that RV pacing was deleterious that catapulted its use.[44–46] The ability to avoid ventricular pacing depends on population and indications,[47,48] and current adult guidelines suggest primarily implanting a biventricular or conduction system pacemaker in those at risk for pacemaker-induced cardiomyopathy expected to have a pacing burden of more than 40%.[49] Nonetheless, for those patients with intermittent AV block and normal function (or a need for limitation of hardware), these algorithms are safe and may be of benefit. In addition, there is some evidence they do save battery, which is of importance for a younger population.[50]

Implantable Cardioverter Defibrillator Features

Avoidance of inappropriate or unnecessary ICD therapy is a priority for all patients requiring defibrillators. Within the adult population, both longer/higher rate detection algorithms and antitachycardia pacing (ATP) reduce shock delivery. Although ventricular arrhythmias in the adult population differ in etiology and rate tolerance compared with those in children, a working knowledge of the adult evidence is of use for the pediatric and ACHD electrophysiologist. In reference to the length/rate of detection, randomized control trials have shown that longer detection times prevent shocks without adverse consequences (such as syncope). In the MADIT-RIT trial, inappropriate therapies were reduced by both increasing rate cutoff to 200 bpm and prolonging time before therapy with rate cutoff 170 bpm. In addition, mortality was reduced in the higher rate therapy group.[51] The ADVANCE III trial showed that longer interval detection times (30–40 intervals vs 18–24 intervals) reduced the rate of ATP delivery, shocks, and inappropriate shocks.[52] These studies and others have been implemented into the programming guidelines that now suggest that, for primary prevention, the

slowest tachycardia therapy zone be programmed between 185 and 200 bpm and that detection times should be at least 6 to 12 seconds or 30 intervals.[53] Although these values should not necessarily be applied directly to all pediatric or ACHD patients, when determining how to program an ICD, it is worth noting that short detection times and slower rate cutoffs may not be of benefit (**Fig. 5**A).

In addition to longer duration/faster rate cutoffs, ATP is useful in terminating ventricular arrhythmia events without shocks (**Fig. 5**B). In the PROVE trial, ATP was able to terminate 93% of episodes in which it was attempted, with low rate of

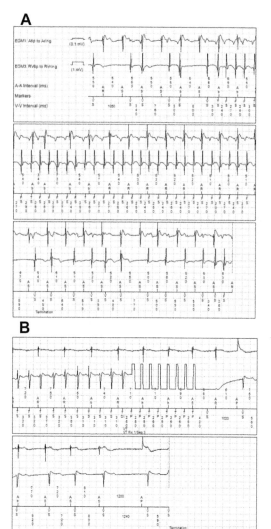

Fig. 5. Modern programming strategies can reduce need for defibrillator shocks. (A) Prolonged detection time allows a self-limited run of ventricular tachycardia to terminate without therapy. (B) In a different patient, ATP terminates a sustained ventricular tachycardia without shock and also without the battery impact of capacitor charging.

acceleration requiring shock.[54] Given the safety and success profile of ATP, adult guidelines now include a class I recommendation of at least 1 ATP attempt with a minimum of 8 stimuli and a cycle length of 84% to 88% of the tachycardia cycle length to reduce total shocks, unless proven ineffective or proarrhythmic.[53]

Remote Monitoring Features

The ability to intervene early during device issues or arrhythmias is a well-known predictor of success. Remote monitoring is now universally available and usage a class I recommendation in pediatric and congenital device therapy.[55] Although the data does show its safety and efficacy in detection of events within the pediatric and ACHD population,[56,57] there is a paucity of data on its effect on overall clinical outcomes. Adult studies have leveraged the high utilization rate of devices to look more closely at how remote monitoring influences mortality and health-care utilization. In a 269,471-person study, Varma and colleagues found that consistent remote monitoring was associated with reduced mortality.[58] In addition, device companies are continuing to develop new algorithms and monitoring techniques, which can help physicians catalog arrhythmia burdens and predict heart failure exacerbations.

SUMMARY

The world of CIED technology is growing and changing rapidly. In addition, with the improvements of cardiac surgery and neonatal care, more children are surviving with congenital heart disease and thus becoming adults who will often have heart rhythm sequelae in their lifetimes. Therefore, the pediatric and congenital electrophysiologist should stay up to date on emerging technology, techniques, and data regarding CIED use. As discussed in this review, technological advancement in CIEDs will remain driven by industry and thus issues relevant to adult patients. Still, it is likely that pediatric/congenital patients will benefit by continued advancements in adult CIED therapy, with creative adaptation where necessary.

CLINICS CARE POINTS

- CIED innovation is largely driven by adult needs. However, many overlapping goals tend to benefit pediatric or ACHD recipients such as reduced device size, and longer battery longevity. Pediatric and ACHD implanters should stay up to date with device development and procedural modifications because they may be of considerable benefit to our patient population.

- Several tools exist to guide lead implantation. The pediatric and ACHD provider may be able to leverage or modify these tools to achieve desired site of lead in small patients or those with complex anatomy.

- Infection following CIED implantation is high risk in pediatrics and may be more likely to occur in patients who have bleeding in the pocket following implant. Given the increased prevalence of children and young adults on anticoagulation and antiplatelet therapy, familiarity with adult protocols for managing anticoagulation around CIED implantation is crucial.

- ICD programming is highly variable in the pediatric and ACHD population. Although adult data cannot be extrapolated exactly to pediatrics, there is good evidence that longer detect times or rate cutoffs may reduce inappropriate therapies while maintaining safety in adults. This data should be considered when programming devices in younger patients.

CONFLICTS OF INTEREST

The authors have no disclosures.

REFERENCES

1. Elmqvest R, Senning A. Implantable pacemaker for the heart. In: Smyth CN, editor. Medical electronics: proceedings of the second international conference on medical electronics, Paris. London, UK: Liffe and Sons; 1959. p. 24–7, 1960:253-254. Abstract.
2. Cohen SI, Zoll P. The pioneer whose discoveries prevent sudden death. Salem (NH): Free People Publishing; 2014. p. 105–11.
3. Cohen SI. On the life of Larry Graves: the first child ever to have a totally implanted pacemaker. Tex Heart Inst J 2016;43(1):7–10.
4. McLeod KA. Cardiac pacing in infants and children. Heart 2010;96(18):1502–8.
5. Greenspon AJ, Patel JD, Lau E, et al. 16 year trends in the infection burden for pacemakers and implantable cardiovert-defibrillators in the United States 1993 to 2008. J Am Coll Cardiol 2011;58:1001–6.
6. Liu P, Zhou Yi-Feng, Yang P, et al. Optimized axillary vein technique versus subclavian vein technique in cardiovascular implantable electronic device implantation: a randomized controlled study. Chin Med J 2016;129(22):2647–51.

7. Kim KH, Park KM, Nam GY, et al. Comparison of the axillary venous approach and subclavian venous approach for efficacy of permanent pacemaker implantation. 8 year-follow-up results. Circ J 2014; 78(4):865–71.

8. Kirkfeldt RE, Johansen JB, Nohr EA, et al. Pneumothorax in cardiac pacing: a population-based cohort study of 28,860 Danish patients. Europace 2012; 14(8):1132–8.

9. Singh HR, Batra AS, Balaji S. Pacing in children. Ann Pediatr Cardiol 2013;6(1):46–51.

10. Yang F, Kulbk G. A new trick to a routine procedure: taking the fear out of the axillary vein stick using the 35-degree caudal view. Europace 2015;17(7):1157–60.

11. Seto AH, Jolly A, Salcedo J. Ultrasound guided venous access for pacemakers and defibrillators. J Cardiovasc Electrophysiol 2013;24(3):370–4.

12. Chandler JK, Apte N, Ranka S, et al. Ultrasound guided axillary vein access: an alternative approach to venous access for cardiac device implantation. J Cardiovasc Electrophysiol 2021;32(2): 458–65.

13. Tagliari AP, Kochi AN, Mastella B, et al. Axillary vein puncture guided by ultrasound vs cephalic vein dissection in pacemaker and defibrillator implant: a multicenter randomized clinical trial. Heart Rhythm 2020;17(9):1554–60.

14. D'Arrigo S, Perna F, Annetta MG, et al. Ultrasound-guided access to the axillary vein for implantation of cardiac implantable electronic devices: a systematic review and meta-analysis. J Vasc Access 2021. https://doi.org/10.1177/11297298211054621. 11297298211054621.

15. Migliore F, Fais L, Vio R, et al. Axillary vein access for permanent pacemaker and implantable cardioverter defibrillator implantation: fluoroscopy compared to ultrasound. Pacing Clin Electrophysiol 2020;43(6): 566–72.

16. Bozyel S, Yalniz A, Aksu T, et al. Ultrasound-guided combined pectoral nerve block and axillary venipuncture for the implantation of cardiac implantable electronic devices. Pacing Clin Electrophysiol 2019; 42:1026–31.

17. Clark BC, Janson CM, Nappo L, et al. Ultrasound-guided axillary venous access for pediatric and adult congenital lead implantation. Pacing Clin Electrophysiol 2019;42(2):166–70.

18. Gongiorni MG, Proclemer A, Dobreanu D, et al. Preferred tools and techniques for implantation of cardiac electronic devices in Europe: results of the European Heart Rhythm Association survey. Europace 2013;15:1664–8.

19. Hasan F, Nedios S, Karosiene Z, et al. Perioperative complications after pacemaker implantation: higher complication rates with subclavian vein puncture than with cephalic vein cutdown. J Intervent Card Electrophysiol 2022;66(4):857–63.

20. Janousek J, Van Geldorp IE, Krupickova S, et al. Permanent cardiac pacing in children: choosing the optimal pacing site. Circulation 2013;127(5): 613–23.

21. Karpawich PP, Singh H, Zelin K. Optimizing paced ventricular function in patients with and without repaired congenital heart disease by contractility-guided lead implant. Pacing Clin Electrophpysiol 2015;38(1):54–62.

22. Sharma AD, Rizo-Patron C, Hallstrom AP, et al. Percent right ventricular pacing predicts outcomes in the DAVID trial. Heart Rhythm 2005;2(8):830–4.

23. Victor F, Mabo P, Mansour H, et al. A randomized comparison of permanent septal versus apical right ventricular pacing: short-term results. J Cardiovasc Electrophysiol 2006;17(3):238–42.

24. Cano O, Osca J, Sancho-Tello MJ, et al. Comparison of effectiveness of right ventricular septal pacing versus right ventricular apical pacing. Am J Cardiol 2010;105(10):1426–32.

25. Mond HG. The road to right ventricular septal pacing: techniques and tools. Pacing Clin Electrophysiol 2010;33(7):888–98.

26. Vinocur JM. Fortuitous left bundle branch area pacing in a small child. JACC Case Rep 2021;3(16): 1730–5.

27. Osmanck P, Stos P, Herman D, et al. The insufficiency of left anterior oblique and the usefulness of right anterior oblique projection for correct localization of a computed tomography-verified right ventricular lead into the midseptum. Circ Arrhythm and Electrophysiol 2013;6(4):719–25.

28. Mond HG, Feldman A, Kumar S. Alternate site right ventricular pacing: defining template scoring. Pacing Clin Electrophysiol 2011;34:1080–6.

29. Chen D, Wei H, Tang Jiao. A randomized comparison of fluoroscopic techniques for implanting pacemaker lead on the right ventricular outflow tract septum. Int J Cardiovasc Imaging 2016;32: 721–8.

30. Das A, Kahali D. Ventricular septal pacing: optimum method to position the lead. Indian Heart J 2018; 70(5):713–20.

31. Squara F, Poulard A, Scarlatti D, et al. New road to septal pacing using patient tailored fluoroscopy criteria: a prospective comparative study of the individualized left anterior oblique projection with caudal angulation. Circ Arrhyth Electrophysiol 2020;13(12).

32. Greenspon AJ, Eby EL, Pertrilla AA, et al. Treatment patterns, costs, and mortality among Medicare beneficiaries with CIED infection. Pacing Clin Electrophyiol 2018;41(5):495.

33. Olsen T, Jorgensen OD, Nielsen JC, et al. Incidence of device-related infection in 97,750 patients: clinical data from the complete Danish device cohort (1982-2018). Eur Heart J 2019;40(23):1862.

34. Link MS, Hill SL, Cliff DI, et al. Comparison of frequency of complications of implantable cardioverter-defibrillators in children versus adults. Am J Cardiol 1999;83(2):263–6.

35. Chen Spenser Y, Ceresnak SR, Montonaga KS, et al. Antibiotic prophylaxis practices in pediatric cardiac implantable electronic device procedures: a survey of the pediatric and congenital electrophysiology society (PACES). Pediatr Cardiol 2018; 39(6):1129–33.

36. Tarakji KG, Mittal S, Kennergren C, et al. Antibacterial envelope to prevent cardiac implantable device infection. N Engl J Med 2019;380(20):1895.

37. Mittal S, Wilkoff BL, Kennergren C, et al. The worldwide randomized antibiotic envelope infection prevention (WRAP-IT) trial: long-term follow up. Heart Rhythm 2020;17(7):1115.

38. Birnie DH, Healey JS, Wells GA, et al. Pacemaker or defibrillator surgery without interruption of anticoagulation. N Engl J Med 2013;368(22):2084.

39. McCrindle BW, Michelson AD, Van Bergen AH, et al. Thromboprophylaxis for children post Fontan procedure: insights from the UNIVERSE study. J Am Heart Assoc 2021;10(22):e021765.

40. Birnie DH, Healey JS, Wells GA, et al. Continued vs. interrupted direct oral anticoagulants at the time of device surgery, in patients with moderate to high risk of arterial thrombo-embolic events (BRUISE CONTROL-2). Eur Heart J 2018;39(44):3973.

41. Notaristefano F, Angeli F, Verdecchia P, et al. Device-pocket hematoma after cardiac implantable electronic devices. Circ Arrhythm Electrophysiol 2020; 13(4):e008372.

42. Essebag V, Healey JS, Joza J, et al. Effect of direct oral anticoagulants, warfarin, and antiplatelet agents on risk of device pocket hematoma: combined analysis of BRUISE CONTROL 1 and 2. Circ Arrhythm Electrophysiol 2019;12(10):3007545.

43. Auricchio A, Ellenbogen KA. Reducing ventricular pacing frequency in patients with atrioventricular block: is it time to change the current pacing paradigm. Circ Arrhythm Electrophysiol 2016;9(9): e004404.

44. Wilkoff BL, Cook JR, Epstein AE, et al. Dual chamber pacing or ventricular backup pacing in patients with an implantable defibrillator: the Dual Chamber and VVI implantable Defibrillator (DAVID) Trial. JAMA 2002;288(24):3115–23.

45. Sweeney MO, Hellkamp AS, Ellenbogen KA, et al. Adverse effect of ventricular pacing on heart failure and atrial fibrillation among patients with normal baseline QRS duration in clinical trial of pacemaker therapy for sinus node dysfunction. Circulation 2003;107(23):2932–7.

46. Casavant DA, Belk P. The story of managed ventricular pacing. J Innov Card Rhythm Manag 2021; 12(8):4625–32.

47. Stockburger M, Boveda S, Moreno J, et al. Long-term clinical effect of ventricular pacing reduction with a changeover mode to minimize ventricular pacing in general pacemaker population. Eur Heart J 2015;36(3):151–7.

48. Boriani G, Tukkie R, Manolis AS, et al. Atrial antitachycardia pacing and managed ventricular pacing in bradycardia patients with paroxysmal or persistent atrial tachyarrhythmias: the MINVERA randomized multicentre international trial. Eur Heart J 2014;35(35):2352–62.

49. Kusumoto FM, Schoenfeld MH, Co Barrnett, et al. 2018 ACC/AHA/HRS guideline on the evaluation and management of patients with bradycardia and cardiac conduction delay: executive summary: a report of the American college of cardiology/American heart association task force on clinical practice guidelines and the heart rhythm society. J Am Coll Cardiol 2019;74(7): 932–87.

50. Stockburger M, Defaye P, Boveda S, et al. Safety and efficiency of ventricular pacing prevention with an AAI-DDD changeover mode in patients with sinus node disease or atrioventricular block: impact on battery longevity-a sub-study of the ANSWER trial. Europace 2016;18(5):739–46.

51. Moss AJ, Schuger C, Beck CA, et al. Reduction in inappropriate therapy and mortality through ICD programming. N Engl J Med 2012;367(24): 2275.

52. Gasparini M, Proclemer A, Klersy C, et al. Effect of long detection interval vs standard detection interval for implantable cardioverter-defibrillators on anti-tachycardia pacing and shock delivery: the ADVANCE III randomized clinical trial. JAMA 2013; 309(18):1903.

53. Wilkoff BL, Fauchier L, Stiles MK, et al. 2015 HRS/EHRA/APHRS/SOLAECE expert consensus statement on optimal implantable cardioverter defibrillator programming and testing. Heart Rhythm 2016;13(2):e50–86.

54. Saeed M, Neason CG, Razavi M, et al. Programming antitachycardia pacing for primary prevention in patients with implantable cardioverter defibrillators: results from the PROVE trial. J Cardiovasc Electrophysiol 2010;21(12):1349.

55. Shah MJ, Silka MJ, Avari Silva JN, et al. PACES expert consensus statement on the indications and management of cardiovascular implantable electronic devices in pediatric patients. Heart Rhythm 2021;18(11):1888–924.

56. Leoni L, Padalino M, Baffanti R, et al. Pacemaker remote monitoring in the pediatric population: is it a real solution? Pacing Clin Electrophysiol 2015; 38(5):565–71.

57. Dechert BE, Serwer GA, Bradley DJ, et al. Cardiac Implantable electronic device remote monitoring

surveillance in pediatric and congenital heart disease: utility relative to frequency. Heart Rhythm 2015;12(1):117–22.

58. Varma J, Piccini JP, Snell J, et al. The relationship between level of adherence to automatic wireless remote monitoring and survival in pacemaker and defibrillator patients. J Am Coll Cardiol 2015; 65(24):2601–10.

59. Du L, Zhang Y, Wang W, et al. Perioperative anticoagulation management in patients on chronic oral anticoagulant therapy undergoing cardiac devices implantation: a meta-analysis. Pacing Clin Electrophysiol 2014;37(11):1573–86.

60. Dandamudi G, Vijayaraman P. How to perform permanent His bundle pacing in routine clinical practice. Heart Rhythm 2016;13(6):1362–6.

Current Device Needs for Patients with Pediatric and Congenital Heart Disease

Heather M. Giacone, MD[a],*, Anne M. Dubin, MD, FHRS[a]

KEYWORDS

• Pacemaker • Pediatric devices • FDA • Congenital heart disease

KEY POINTS

- There are currently no pacemakers or internal cardioverter defibrillators that are Food and Drug Administration (FDA)-labeled for use in pediatric population (<18 years of age).
- Pediatric and congenital heart disease patients are at higher risk of cardiac implantable electronic device-related complications, in part due to off-label use.
- Collaboration among the FDA, industry, and pediatric societies has led to new strategies to advance pediatric devices.

CASE VIGNETTE

A 31-week gestation, 2.0 kg infant was delivered emergently due to fetal complete heart block associated with hydrops and a ventricular escape rate of 47 bpm. Postnatally, pacing was required emergently. There was concern that implantation of a traditional permanent epicardial pacemaker system would result in skin erosion due to anasarca and decreased skin integrity in a premature infant. After a full discussion with the family, and with emergent local institutional review board approval and emergency use authorization from the Food and Drug Administration (FDA) under the Expanded Access Medical Device pathway, this patient underwent placement of a 25-cm epicardial bipolar ventricular lead (Medtronic CapSure Epi model 4968) and the novel implantable pacing generator (Medtronic MC1VR01 Micra Leadless Pacing System VR TCP with a Pediatric implantable pulse generator header) placed in a subrectus pocket (**Fig. 1**), as previously reported by Berul and colleagues for use as a permanent epicardial system.[1]

This case illustrates a multitude of unique considerations for pediatric patients undergoing device implantations including small patient size; availability of current devices not specifically designed for pediatric patients; counseling parents on alternative uses of devices; and long-term considerations of pacemakers in children due to life-long pacing dependency. Pacemaker implantation options for neonates less than 2.5 kg are extremely limited, secondary to a significant mismatch of patient and generator size.[1] There have been several novel approaches to pacemaker therapy in the smallest infants including implantation of temporary epicardial pacing wires to allow for patient growth before permanent epicardial pacemaker implantation or placement of a permanent epicardial lead to an externalized generator. Both approaches are not ideal as they are temporizing at best and require a subsequent procedure in the first few months of life. They also increase the risk of infection in a compromised neonate.

Current State of Pediatric Device Therapy

In a recent survey, 96% of pediatric electrophysiologists believe that there is a deficit in cardiac

a Department of Pediatric Cardiology, Lucile Packard Children's Hospital at Stanford University, 750 Welch Road, Palo Alto, CA 94304, USA
* Corresponding author.
E-mail address: hgiacone@stanford.edu

Card Electrophysiol Clin 15 (2023) 527–534
https://doi.org/10.1016/j.ccep.2023.06.005

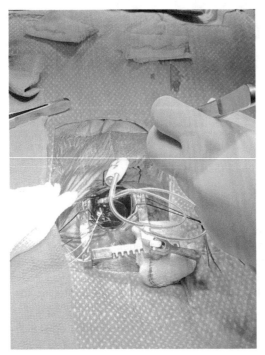

Fig. 1. Surgical implantation of a 25-cm epicardial bipolar ventricular lead (Medtronic Capsure Epi model 4968) and the novel implantable pacing generator (Medtronic MC1VR01 Micra Leadless Pacing System VR TCP) with a Pediatric implantable pulse generator header.

implantable electronic devices (CIEDs) that are appropriate for pediatric patients or FDA-labeled specifically for pediatric use.[2] Although there are many FDA-approved CIEDs currently used in the pediatric population, none are specifically designed for pediatric patients, and few undergo rigorous testing in the pediatric population. Currently, the total number of pediatric patients with CIEDs makes up less than 1% to 2% of total CIED implantations.[3,4] Although this is a small percentage currently, the number of pediatric and congenital heart disease (CHD) patients with device needs is growing and pediatric-specific devices will be in even higher demand in the next decade.[5] Moderate to severe CHD occurs in 6 out of 1000 live births, many of which have tachyarrhythmias or bradyarrhythmias associated with their native anatomy or as sequelae of surgical procedures which require CIEDs for management.[6] Survival estimates for these patients have increased from 25% expected survival to adulthood in the 1960s to over 90% survival to adulthood in the current era.[7] Many of these patients will require several decades of pacing therapy. Therefore, there is a growing population of pediatric and CHD patients who require device implantations yet have few CIED devices designed, or safety tested for them.

Challenges of Pediatric Patients

Overview

Pediatric/CHD patients who require CIED implantation comprise an extremely heterogenous population making CIED device design a difficult target. Complex intracardiac anatomy and small vascular size and/or abnormalities can complicate pacemaker placement. Small patient size, somatic growth issues, and the need for life-long pacing should be considered before device placement and will alter the type of device used.[8–11] Although the CIED type chosen for implantation is largely based on the above patient characteristics, surgical expertise and local resources also influence decision-making.[9,11,12]

Patient size and somatic growth

Patient size, as demonstrated in our case described above, often limits CIED options. Smaller vascular diameters can have a higher incidence of venous occlusion,[11,13] although some studies indicate that venous occlusion may be multifactorial.[14] Nonetheless, transvenous CIED implantation is not routinely performed in young or small patients given the potentially life-long need for pacing. There is also an increased risk of pacemaker generator erosion with the smallest of patients.[13] Although there is much practice variation, most centers will regularly wait until a patient is 10 to 15 kg before performing a transvenous CIED implantation. In a recent international survey addressing lowest acceptable weight of patients undergoing transvenous CIED implantation, 45% of centers reported 10 to 20 kg, whereas 29% of centers waited until patients were 20 to 30 kg, and 9% waited until patients were over 30 kg.[12] Although successful implantation of transvenous CIEDs has been reported in patients less than 10 to 15 kg, this is not the standard of care in most institutions.[11,13–16] The innovation of leadless pacemakers overcomes the risk of vascular occlusion, but unfortunately the large delivery sheath system (27F), difficult septal positioning due to small cardiac size, and limited long-term retrieval options make this innovation currently suboptimal for most pediatric patients. Implantation of a leadless pacemaker has been successfully reported in pediatric patients as small as 25 kg, although difficulty positioning onto the cardiac septum was noted.[17] When transvenous lead implantation is not appropriate in patients requiring internal cardioverter defibrillator (ICD) implantation, non-traditional ICD lead implantation locations can be used including subcutaneous, thoracic, or pericardiac, but these are associated with higher lead fracture rates.[18]

In addition, somatic growth trajectory of pediatric patients needs to be considered when choosing CIED type. Excess lead length, or lead slack, is provided to the patient during both epicardial and endocardial CIED implantations to account for expected somatic growth and to increase the potential longevity of leads by decreasing risk of failure or fracture with inadequate lead length.[19,20] It is reported that during rapid somatic growth, patients can use 10 mm/y of lead slack in transvenous systems.[19] Epicardial devices can provide more room for lead slack.

Longevity of pacing need and location of ventricular pacing

Many pediatric patients who require CIED implantation are device-dependent for the remainder of their lives.[9] Even with the most current devices and longer lasting batteries, serial procedures are required which place the patient at higher risk of morbidities or mortality during subsequent surgeries.[11,13] In pediatric or young adult patients who present with endovascular lead failures, lead extraction and subsequent replacement instead of lead abandonment is highly considered when possible due to the long-term need for vascular patency. Of course, a risk–benefit analysis for each patient is made as current reported major complications for lead extractions is approximately 1% with each extraction.[21,22]

Chronic ventricular pacing burden should also be considered when deciding on the type of CIED implantation in pediatric and CHD patients due to the risk of potential pacing induced cardiomyopathy. Single-site right ventricle (RV) pacing has been reported to place certain types of CHD patients at higher risk for pacing induced cardiomyopathy, therefore when able, apical pacing or multisite ventricular pacing to provide resynchronization during epicardial implantation is preferred for patients with single-ventricle physiology, double outlet right ventricle, atrioventricular canal defects, and transposition of the great arteries (d-transposition of the great arteries [d-TGA] and congenitally corrected TGA).[23,24] In addition, if the patient is pacemaker-dependent, biventricular or multisite ventricular pacing via an epicardial system should be considered to decrease the rate of sudden cardiac death due to acute lead failure with only single site ventricular pacing leads.[25]

Congenital heart disease

Improvements in medical and surgical management have improved survival in patients with CHD. This survival, however, is complicated by short- and long-term sequelae including bradyarrhythmias and tachyarrhythmias which may require medical and device therapy. These patients can have an inherent risk of heart block or develop heart block following surgical procedure.[26] They can be at risk of atrial and ventricular tachyarrhythmias which can lead to sudden death.[27] Thus, patients with CHD often require CIED placement at some point in their lives.

Device therapy in this population is often complicated by inherent structural abnormalities. These can include systemic right ventricles, single ventricles, or intracardiac shunts which can preclude the "typical" transvenous CIED placement. Intracardiac shunting is considered a contraindication for a transvenous approach secondary to the increased risk of paradoxic emboli and stroke.[9,28] Patients with atrial switch surgery (Mustard or Senning procedure) for TGA often develop occlusion or leaks of the atrial baffle which can limit the lead size/type for CIED placement. Finally, patients with single-ventricle physiology may require an extracardiac Fontan procedure resulting in direct connection of the superior vena cava (SVC) and inferior vena cava (IVC) to the pulmonary arteries, completely bypassing the heart and making a typical transvenous system impossible.

CHD patients can also have intrinsic or acquired abnormalities of their vasculature. CHD has an increased association of left SVC.[29,30] Patients can develop vascular occlusion secondary to indwelling lines in the postoperative period. With these considerations, it is no surprise that patients with complex CHD are more likely to undergo epicardial CIED implantation compared with those with simple or moderate CHD.[31]

Heart rate considerations

CIED software algorithms were designed for adult patients with lower baseline intrinsic heart rates.[8] Higher baseline intrinsic heart rates, which are physiologic in pediatric patients, can lead to an overall shorter battery life, requiring more frequent generator changes.[32] High heart rates associated with exercise can also lead to inappropriate ICD discharges in the pediatric population.[33] Limitations on rate adaptive atrioventricular (AV) delay settings can lead to pediatric patients reaching upper tracking rate behaviors such as pacemaker Wenckebach during sinus tachycardia. Last, generators with accelerometer-guided rate response technology were designed for implantation in standard infraclavicular locations, which may not be ideal for pediatric or CHD patients with abdominal generators.[8]

Pediatric and Congenital Heart Disease Populations Have Higher Cardiac Implantable Electronic Devices Complication Rates

Both short- and long-term complication rates are higher in pediatric and CHD patients compared with adults receiving CIEDs. Higher periprocedural complication rates are seen in the CHD population compared with the general population (10.6% vs 5.2%).[31] Examples of these complications include lead dysfunction, bleeding, infection, and pneumothorax. Pacemaker implantation in the pediatric population is an independent predictor of late complications such as primary lead failure.[31] ICD complications are also higher in the pediatric population.[5] Inappropriate ICD discharges are higher in both pediatric (21%–25%) and CHD populations (21%–26%) when compared with adult cohorts (10%).[32,34,35] This is attributable to lead failure, t-wave oversensing, or tachycardia (sinus tachycardia or supraventricular tachycardia) reaching heart rate criteria for arrhythmia treatment.[33,34]

Epicardial leads demonstrate decreased overall longevity compared with transvenous leads (76.4% lead survival vs 96.5% at 12 years post-implantation)[36] and failures of epicardial leads are more common (21% vs 6%, respectively, although steroid eluting epicardial leads demonstrate similar survival to transvenous leads).[20] The complete removal of epicardial leads can be difficult due to fibrosis, and many times these leads are capped and abandoned. This does not usually result in any harm to the patient, but cardiac strangulation or coronary compression (5% incidence) has been reported.[37,38] Epicardial systems and abandoned epicardial leads are relative contraindications to MRI that can limit future imaging options.[9,39]

Off-Label Device Use

The vast majority of cardiac devices used in children are used off-label.[8,40] At present, no pacemaker or defibrillator has been approved for use in children less than 18 years by FDA; Micra is approved over age 18 (**Table 1**). Thus, CIEDs implanted are used in an off-label fashion with the result that the device design was not optimum for pediatric patients and clinical studies defining safety and outcome data may not represent the pediatric or CHD populations.[8,40] Currently, there is no formal reporting method of device performance and safety outcomes when FDA-approved devices are used off-label, creating an environment in which safety concerns may not be identified in a timely manner.[40]

Barriers to Development of a Pediatric-Specific Device

Pediatric device development has been slow for a variety of reasons. The population is an extremely heterogenous one with varied structural disease processes which makes traditional clinical trials difficult. There is also a limited financial incentive to investing in the development of a pediatric-specific device, which represents less than 2% of the device market. Finally, there are added technical hurdles to miniaturizing devices. A good example of this is the Sprint Fidelis ICD lead (Medtronic), which was a small 6.6 mm transvenous ICD lead released in 2004. This lead was quickly discovered to have a higher than expected failure rate leading to a recall in 2007.[41] The patients most at risk with this lead were younger patients with higher heart rates and higher activity rates.[8]

Food and Drug Administration-Approval Process for Pediatric Medical Devices

Traditionally, FDA approval requires preclinical and clinical testing via the pre-market application (PMA) pathway to demonstrate a risk–benefit profile and ultimately determine safety and efficacy. This is usually achieved via multiple randomized control trials, which often are not possible in the small pediatric population. Recognizing this circumstance, FDA has developed other potential pathways for device approval which are more applicable to the pediatric and CHD populations.

The Human Device Exemption (HDE) pathway was created to specifically address the use of devices in those with rare diseases (<4000 cases per year). Under the HDE pathway, there must be evidence of *probable benefit* and that this benefit outweighs any risk of illness or injury as well as proof that unreasonable risks are not present. Clinical data suitable for the HDE pathway can include a single-arm clinical trial with controls represented by retrospective data.[8] The HDE pathway is feasible for devices used in smaller populations such as pediatric and CHD device implantations. Cardiac devices have been approved for use in pediatric CHD populations using the HDE pathway (ie, Berlin Heart EXCOR® ventricular-assist device), but currently, there are not any CIED devices approved in this manner[40] (see **Table 1**).

The 510(k) pathway is restricted to devices that are classified as low risk to patients (Class I) or moderate risk (Class II devices, such as cardiac monitors), but cannot be used for high-risk devices (Class III) such as pacemakers and ICDs.[40] This pathway has been used to obtain FDA approval of the Medtronic LINQ II™ Insertable Cardiac Monitor for pediatric use (see **Table 1**).

Table 1
Cardiac medical devices approved for use in pediatric or sub-pediatric populations

Medical Device	Age Included in Studies for Approval or FDA Age Specification on Approval	Fiscal Year Approved	FDA Pathway
Freezor and Freezor Xtra Cardiac Cryoablation Catheters; Medtronic Inc	Pediatric	2003,[a] 2022	PMA
LINQ II™ Insertable Cardiac Monitor; Medtronic Inc	>2 year old	2022	501(k)
AMPLATZER PFO Occluder: St Jude Medical Inc	18–60 year old	2017	PMA
AED Plus (Defibrillator); Zoll Medical Corporation	>2 year old	2017	PMA
HeartSine Samaritan PAD 350P (SAM350P), HeartSine Samaritan PAD 360P (SAM360P) HeartSine Smaritan PAD 450P (SM450P)- (Defibrillator); HeartSine Technologies LLC	>1 year old	2017	PMA
Melody Transcatheter Pulmonary Valve (TPV) and Ensemble/Ensemble II Transcatheter Valve Delivery System; Medtronic Inc	Pediatric	2017	PMA
Micra Transcatheter Pacing System (MC1VR01 and Programmer Application Software Model SW022 Version 1.1); Medtronic Inc	>18 year old	2016	PMA
LifeVest Wearable Defibrillator; ZOLL Manufacturing Corporation	18 and younger	2015	PMA
EXCOR® Pediatric Ventricular Assist Device; Berlin Heart Inc	Pediatric	2017	HDE
The Edwards SAPIAN XT Transcatheter Heart Valve (THV); Edwards Lifesciences, LLC	Pediatric and Adult	2016	PMA
Blazer Open-Irrigated Ablation Catheter; Boston Scientific Corp	18 and older	2016	PMA
Medtronic Melody Transcatheter Pulmonary Valve (Model PB10) and Medtronic Ensemble Transcatheter Valve Delivery System (NU10)	Pediatric	2010	HDE
Impella RP system: Abiomed Inc	Pediatric with clinical specifications	2015, 2017	HDE
CONTEGRA Pulmonary Valved Conduit: Medtronic Inc	Pediatric	2003	HDE

Bold indicates electrophysiologic-specific devices.
Abbreviations: PFO, patent foramen ovale; AED, automated external defibrillator.
[a] Received approval to expand indication to pediatric patients in 2022.
Information obtained from the following sources: https://www.fda.gov/media/128659/download, https://www.fda.gov/media/107294/download.

Although these alternative pathways can help with device labeling in children, often the difficulties associated with enrolling and performing clinical trials in pediatric and CHD populations limit a company's interest in pursuing pediatric labeling. To address this, there have been multiple initiatives that target strategies for data collection to support FDA applications. In 2007, the FDA Amendments Act allowed the use of post-market data registries to help characterize the risk–benefit profile of devices currently used in an off-label fashion.[8,42] One product of this amendment was the Sentinel system, which is an FDA national electronic system that partners with health care organizations to compile anonymous data and outcomes regarding FDA-approved drugs and devices.[42] The Twenty-first Century Cures Act (2016) emphasizes the use of real-world evidence to underpin regulatory decision-making for medical devices.[43,44] Large clinical registries, which are widely used in pediatric CHD research currently, could be used to obtain real-world data that will better define risk–benefit and outcome profiles of CIEDs within pediatric CHD populations. This registry information would be important not only to potentially support FDA approval in new clinical applications, but also to provide a method of surveillance of safety outcomes because there is no formalized reporting method of devices used in an off-label format.[8-] There has also been initial work assessing the role of computational modeling and simulation techniques to help test design modifications of current CIEDs adjusted for the pediatric/CHD population.[8]

The Center for Devices and Radiological Health (CDRH) Early Feasibility Study (EFS) program is a way to promote device innovation of new devices or modification of a current marketed device while only needing a small number of study participants.[35] The EFS pathway requires smaller numbers of patients for initial testing and allows for device iteration throughout the study.[45] In 2012, the EFS program allowed for the reporting of safety data through clinical use studies. With only small numbers needed (<15) at investigational sites, this provides a more obtainable data set in our small population allowing for regulatory processes and review and early FDA involvement in pediatric device development.

Medical Device Development Advocacy Efforts

The number of pediatric-specific FDA-approved devices remains low. The FDA annually publishes a public summary of the pediatric-specific devices that obtained FDA approval by HDE or PMA pathways in a report to Congress in accordance with 515A(a) (3) of the Food Drug and Cosmetic Act. From fiscal year 2008 to 2017, 447 medical devices have been approved via PMA and HDE pathways. Ninety-six (21%) were approved for use in a pediatric population or pediatric subpopulation, and only 5 for pediatric electrophysiology indications.[46]

Fortunately, advocacy for the pediatric and CHD population with CIEDs has brought awareness to the stark need for pediatric and CHD-specific advancements.[8] Discussions of how to enact reform and bring innovation to this population have started with collaboration among FDA, industry, and the international Pediatric and Congenital Electrophysiology Society (PACES).

FDAs CDRH support regulatory programs for special populations such as pediatric CHD patients to aid in the increased safety of devices.[8] As mentioned above, FDA has been developing innovative new strategies to address the challenges posed by a small pediatric population. Workshops and grants via the Pediatric Device Consortium program and guidance documents have been presented as additional solution options to improve the current scene.[43]

In 2016, PACES, created a task force with a goal to increase collaboration among care providers, industry, and FDA to aid in the development of pediatric EP devices, data, and education. This task force has aided in bringing awareness of the needs of pediatric electrophysiologists and their patients. This collaboration resulted in the pediatric labeling of the Freezor Xtra cardiac cryoablation catheter (Medtronic) using preexisting studies and real-world data.

SUMMARY AND FUTURE DIRECTIONS

The pediatric electrophysiology community believes that there is a paucity of pediatric-specific CIEDs available for their patients.[1,2,8] Although the pediatric and CHD populations requiring CIED implantation are growing, patient size, intracardiac anatomy, expected somatic growth, and longevity of pacing limit the types of CIED implants that can be used. Currently, these populations demonstrate a higher risk of CIED-related complications. The need for CIED advancements has resulted in the establishment of a collaborative forum among the FDA, industry, and pediatric societies to advocate for improvement in the current market for pediatric and CHD-specific devices.

CLINICS CARE POINTS

- Considerations about intracardiac anatomy, need for future surgical procedures, patient size and longevity of pacing need should be

- evaluated before cardiac implantable electronic device (CIED) implantation in the pediatric and congenital heart disease population.

- Currently, there are no CIEDs that are specifically developed and Food and Drug Administration (FDA)-approved for use in the pediatric population. Therefore, CIEDs originally engineered for an adult population, including algorithms and device sizes, can lead to increased complication rates in the pediatric population.

- There is an ongoing collaborative among the FDA, industry and pediatric societies to advance the current pediatric and CHD-specific CIED market.

DISCLOSURES

The authors have nothing to disclose.

REFERENCES

1. Berul CI, Dasgupta S, LeGras MD, et al. Creative concepts: tiny pacemakers for tiny babies. Heart Rhythm 2023;S1547-5271(23):00201–11.

2. Dubin AM, Bar-Cohen YS, Berul CI, et al. Pediatric electrophysiology device needs: a survey from the pediatric and congenital electrophysiology society taskforce on pediatric-specific devices. J Am Heart Assoc 2022;11(22):e026904.

3. McLeod KA. Cardiac pacing in infants and children. Heart 2010;96:1502–8.

4. Epstein AE, DiMarco JP, Ellenbogen KA, et al. American college of cardiology/American heart association task force on practice guidelines (writing committee to revise the ACC/AHA/NASPE 2002 guideline update for implantation of cardiac pacemakers and antiarrhythmia devices); American association for thoracic surgery; society of thoracic surgeons. ACC/AHA/HRS 2008 guidelines for device-based therapy of cardiac rhythm abnormalities: a report of the American college of cardiology/American heart association task force on practice guidelines (writing committee to revise the ACC/AHA/NASPE 2002 guideline update for implantation of cardiac pacemakers and antiarrhythmia devices) developed in collaboration with the American association for thoracic surgery and society of thoracic surgeons. J Am Coll Cardiol 2008;51(21):e1–62. Erratum in: J Am Coll Cardiol. 2009;53(16):1473. Erratum in: J Am Coll Cardiol. 2009;53(1):147.

5. Czosek RJ, Meganathan K, Anderson JB, et al. Cardiac rhythm devices in the pediatric population: utilization and complications. Heart Rhythm 2012;9(2):199–208.

6. Hoffman JIE, Kaplan S, Liberthson RR. Prevalence of congenital heart disease. Am Heart J 2004;147:425–39.

7. Warnes CA. The adult with congenital heart disease: born to be bad? J Am Coll Cardiol 2005;4(1):1–8.

8. Dubin AM, Cannon BC, Saarel EV, et al. Pediatric and congenital electrophysiology society initiative on device needs in pediatric electrophysiology. Heart Rhythm 2019;16:39–46.

9. Shah MJ, Silka MJ, Silva JNA, et al. 2021 PACES expert consensus statement on the indications and management of cardiovascular implantable electronic devices in pediatric patients. Heart Rhythm 2021;18(11):1888–924.

10. Takeuchi D, Tomizawa Y. Pacing device therapy in infants and children: a review. J Artif Organs 2013;16:23–33.

11. Wilhelm BJ, Thöne M, El-Scheich T, et al. Complications and risk assessment of 25 Years in pediatric pacing. Ann Thorac Surg 2015;100(1):147–53.

12. Gonzalez Corcia MC, Cohen MI, Paul T, et al. Preliminary assessment of paediatric electrophysiology cardiac implantable electronic device resources around the world. Cardiol Young 2022;32(12):1989–93.

13. Vos LM, Kammeraad JAE, Freund MW, et al. Long-term outcome of transvenous pacemaker implantation in infants: a retrospective cohort study. J.Europace 2017;19(4):581–7.

14. Bar-Cohen Y, Berul CI, Alexander ME, et al. Age, size, and lead factors alone do not predict venous obstruction in children and young adults with transvenous lead systems. Journal Cardiovascular Electrophysiology 2006;17:754–9.

15. Campos-Quintero A, García-Montes JA, Cruz-Arias R, et al. Endocardial pacing in infants and young children weighing less than 10 kilograms. Rev Esp Cardiol 2018;71(1):48–51.

16. Wildbolz M, Dave H, Weber R, et al. Pacemaker implantation in neonates and infants: favorable outcomes with epicardial pacing systems. Pediatr Cardiol 2020;41(5):910–7.

17. Breatnach CR, Dunne L, Al-Alawi K, et al. Leadless Micra pacemaker use in the pediatric population: device implantation and short-term outcomes. Pediatr Cardiol 2020;41(4):683–6.

18. Radbill AE, Triedman JK, Berul CI, et al. System survival of nontransvenous implantable cardioverter-defibrillators compared to transvenous implantable cardioverter-defibrillators in pediatric and congenital heart disease patients. Heart Rhythm 2010;7(2):193–8.

19. Gheissari A, Hordof AJ, Spotnitz HM. Transvenous pacemakers in children: relation of lead length to anticipated growth. Ann Thorac Surg 1991;52(1):118–21.

20. Silvetti MS, Drago F, Grutter G, et al. Twenty years of paediatric cardiac pacing: 515 pacemakers and 480 leads implanted in 292 patients. Europace 2006;8(7):530–6.

21. Fender EA, Killu AM, Cannon BC, et al. Lead extraction outcomes in patients with congenital heart disease. Europace 2017;19(3):441–6.

22. Kusumoto FM, Schoenfeld MH, Wilkoff BL, et al. 2017 HRS expert consensus statement on cardiovascular implantable electronic device lead management and extraction. Heart Rhythm 2017;14(12):e503–51.

23. Bulic A, Zimmerman FJ, Ceresnak SR, et al. Ventricular pacing in single ventricles-A bad combination. Heart Rhythm 2017;14(6):853–7.

24. Balaji S, Sreeram N. The development of pacing induced ventricular dysfunction is influenced by the underlying structural heart defect in children with congenital heart disease. Indian Heart J 2017; 69(2):240–3.

25. Ceresnak SR, Perera JL, Motonaga KS, et al. Ventricular lead redundancy to prevent cardiovascular events and sudden death from lead fracture in pacemaker-dependent children. Heart Rhythm 2015;12(1):111–6.

26. Romer AJ, Tabbutt S, Etheridge SP, et al. Atrioventricular block after congenital heart surgery: analysis from the pediatric cardiac critical care Consortium. J Thorac Cardiovasc Surg 2019;157(3):1168–77.e2.

27. Khairy P, Silka MJ, Moore JP, et al. Sudden cardiac death in congenital heart disease. Eur Heart J 2022;43(22):2103–15.

28. Khairy P, Landzberg MJ, Gatzoulis MA, et al. Epicardial versus Endocardial pacing and Thromboembolic events Investigators. Transvenous pacing leads and systemic thromboemboli in patients with intracardiac shunts: a multicenter study. Circulation 2006;113(20):2391–7.

29. Shiekh Eldin G, El-Segaier M, Galal MO. High prevalence rate of left superior vena cava determined by echocardiography in patients with congenital heart disease in Saudi Arabia. Libyan J Med 2013;8(1): 21679.

30. Albay S, Cankal F, Kocabiyik N, et al. Double superior vena cava. Morphologie 2006;90(288):39–42.

31. Opić P, van Kranenburg M, Yap SC, et al. Complications of pacemaker therapy in adults with congenital heart disease: a multicenter study. Int J Cardiol 2013;168(4):3212–6.

32. Stanner C, Horndasch M, Vitanova K, et al. Neonates and infants requiring life-long cardiac pacing: how reliable are epicardial leads through childhood? Int J Cardiol 2019;15(297):43–8.

33. Garnreiter JM. Inappropriate ICD shocks in pediatric and congenital heart disease patients. J Innov Card Rhythm Manag 2017;8(11):2898–906.

34. Berul CI, Van Hare GF, Kertesz NJ. Results of a multicenter retrospective implantable cardioverter-defibrillator registry of pediatric and congenital heart disease patients. J Am Coll Cardiol 2008;51:1685–91.

35. Nishii N, Noda T, Nitta T, et al. Risk factors for the first and second inappropriate implantable cardioverter-defibrillator therapy. Int J Cardiol Heart Vasc 2021; 34:100779.

36. Medtronic. Medtronic lead performance reports: epicardial lead 4968 CapSure Epi and endovenous lead 5086 CapSureFix Novus at 12 years. Available from https://wwwp.medtronic.com/product performance/model/5086MRI-capsurefix-novus-mri.html and https://wwwp.medtronic.com/product-performance/model/4968-capsure-epi.html.

37. Takeuchi D, Tomizawa Y. Cardiac strangulation from epicardial pacemaker leads: diagnosis, treatment, and prevention. Gen Thorac Cardiovasc Surg 2015;63(1):22–9.

38. Mah DY, Prakash A, Porras D, et al. Coronary artery compression from epicardial leads: more common than we think. Heart Rhythm 2018;15(10):1439–47.

39. Ian Paterson D, White JA, Butler CR, Connelly KA, Guerra PG, Hill MD, James MT, Kirpalani A, Lydell CP, Roifman I, Sarak B, Sterns LD, Verma A, Wan D, Secondary Panel, Crean AM, Grosse-Wortmann L, Hanneman K, Leipsic J, Manlucu J, Nguyen ET, Sandhu RK, Villemaire C, Wald RM, Windram J. 2021 update on safety of magnetic resonance imaging: joint statement from Canadian cardiovascular society/Canadian society for cardiovascular magnetic resonance/Canadian heart rhythm society. Can J Cardiol 2021;37(6):835–47.

40. Almond CS. The FDA review process for cardiac medical devices in children: a review for the clinician. Prog Pediatric Cardiology 2012;33:105–9.

41. Atallah J, Erickson CC, Cecchin F, et al. Pediatric and Congenital Electrophysiology Society (PACES). Multi-institutional study of implantable defibrillator lead performance in children and young adults: results of the Pediatric Lead Extractability and Survival Evaluation (PLEASE) study. Circulation 2013; 127(24):2393–402.

42. Avorn J, Kesselheim A, Sarpatwari A. The FDA amendments act of 2007 - assessing its effects a decade later. N Engl J Med 2018;379(12):1097–9.

43. Ibrahim N, Gillette N, Patel H, et al. Regulatory science, and how device regulation will shape our future. Pediatr Cardiol 2020;41:469–74.

44. US Department of Health and Human Services, Food and Drug Administration, Center for Devices and Radiological Health, Center for Biologics Evaluation and Research. Use of Real-World Evidence to Support Regulatory Decision-Making for Medical Devices - Guidance for Industry and Food and Drug Administration Staff 2017.

45. Investigational Device Exemptions (IDEs) for Early Feasibility Medical Device Clinical Studies, Including Certain First in Human (FIH) Studies (2013) U.S. Department of Health and Human Services, Food and Drug Administration, Center for Devices and Radiological Health, Center for Biologics Evaluation Research., Silver Spring.

46. Food and Drug Administration. Report to Congress: Annual Report Premarket Approval of Pediatric Uses of Devices. FY2017. Obtained from https://www.fda.gov/media/128659/download.

Moving?

Make sure your subscription moves with you!

To notify us of your new address, find your **Clinics Account Number** (located on your mailing label above your name), and contact customer service at:

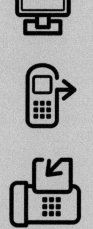

Email: journalscustomerservice-usa@elsevier.com

800-654-2452 (subscribers in the U.S. & Canada)
314-447-8871 (subscribers outside of the U.S. & Canada)

Fax number: 314-447-8029

Elsevier Health Sciences Division
Subscription Customer Service
3251 Riverport Lane
Maryland Heights, MO 63043

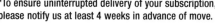

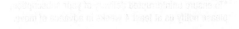

Printed and bound by CPI Group (UK) Ltd, Croydon, CR0 4YY

03/10/2024

01040367-0010